The

NURSING MOTHER'S

Quick Reference Guide and Planner

Essential
Breastfeeding Information
for Mothers with New Babies

KATHLEEN HUGGINS

HARVARD
COMMON
PRESS

© 2020 Quarto Publishing Group USA Inc.
Text © 2015, 2020 Kathleen Huggins

First Published in 2020 by The Harvard Common Press, an imprint of The Quarto Group, 100 Cummings Center, Suite 265-D, Beverly, MA 01915, USA.
T (978) 282-9590 F (978) 283-2742 QuartoKnows.com

The Harvard Common Press titles are also available at discount for retail, wholesale, promotional, and bulk purchase. For details, contact the Special Sales Manager by email at specialsales@quarto.com or by mail at The Quarto Group, Attn: Special Sales Manager, 100 Cummings Center, Suite 265-D, Beverly, MA 01915, USA.

24 23 22 21 20   1 2 3 4 5

ISBN: 978-1-55832-979-9

Digital edition published in 2020

The content for this book appeared in the previously published *The Nursing Mother's Companion, 7th Edition* (The Harvard Common Press 2018).

Library of Congress Cataloging-in-Publication Data available

Design: Sporto
Cover llustration and Illustrations: Gayle Isabelle Ford

Printed in China

CONTENTS

INTRODUCTION

SINCE THE BEGINNING OF HUMANKIND, women have put their infants to breast. Extending the physical bond that begins at conception, they have nourished and protected their young with their bodies. These tender moments, in return, have brought pleasure and fulfillment to the task of mothering. If you are now pregnant, you are probably looking forward to the time in which you will nourish, comfort, and protect your child in the same way as others before you—at the breast.

Perhaps you already feel committed to the idea of nursing. For you, there is no question that you'll breastfeed your baby. Or perhaps, like many women, you have some uncertainties but still feel it's worth a try. Your outlook depends on many things—the value you place on breastfeeding, how your partner feels about it, how your friends have fed their babies, your lifestyle, and your feelings about yourself and your body.

You probably also have some notions about what nursing will be like. Perhaps you think it will be easy and convenient. Maybe you worry that it might not fit in with your activities and plans. You may have concerns about your ability to nurse. Probably you know of other women who tried to nurse but soon gave up. Whatever your attitudes, expectations, and concerns about breastfeeding, these may become powerful determinants in your ultimate success or failure to nurse your baby happily.

IS BREASTFEEDING REALLY BETTER?

You may be under the impression that the decision to breastfeed or bottle-feed is simply a matter of personal preference. Don't let anyone fool you into believing that breast milk and formula are equally good—they are not. Without a doubt, mother's milk alone promotes optimum health and development for babies. It is uniquely designed to meet the complete nutritional needs of the growing human infant. It also protects the infant against illness throughout the entire first year and beyond, as long as nursing continues. Artificial human milk, whether made from cow's milk or soybeans, will never be able to duplicate nature's formula.

Although they do grow on processed infant formulas, babies, like all young mammals, do best with milk from their own species. Human milk contains proteins that promote brain development. In contrast, cow's milk contains proteins that favor muscular growth. The nutritional properties of breast milk are designed for babies' specific growth and developmental needs. Formula manufacturers are continually challenged to include all of the nutrients in breast milk that scientists are gradually identifying as important to infant growth and development.

In recent years, for example, formula manufacturers have acknowledged that the fatty acids in breast milk are necessary to babies' intellectual, motor, and visual development. Now 90 percent of formula in the United States includes ARA and DHA (arachidonic acid and docosahexaenoic acid) made from fermented microalgae and soil fungus. These lab-produced chemicals are meant to substitute for the omega-3 and omega-6 fatty acids that are naturally found in breast milk. When formula manufacturers started adding ARA and DHA to their products, says Marsha Walker, executive director of the National Alliance for Breastfeeding Advocacy, the price of formula immediately rose by 30 percent. Research has shown little evidence for the companies' claims of beneficial effects on brain and eye development, but we do know that some infants suffer from diarrhea and other side effects after drinking these formulas.

Human milk differs from formula, too, in that it contains specific immunities against human illness. In contrast, cow's milk contains specific immunities against bovine disease. For this and other reasons, babies on a formula diet are at greater risk for illness and hospitalization. Diarrheal infections and respiratory illnesses, including respiratory syncytial virus (RSV) are more frequent and serious among these babies. (RSV is the most common cause of pneumonia and bronchiolitis—inflammation of the small airways in the lung—in children younger than one year of age in the United States.) Formula-fed babies develop many more ear infections, which may lead to later speech and reading problems. Urinary tract infections and bacterial meningitis are also more common among artificially fed infants.

Although most parents don't know this, powdered formula is not sterile. Besides lacking the anti-infective components of breast milk, powdered formula may be contaminated with bacteria (*Cronobacter spp.*, formerly known as *Enterobacter sakazakii*) that can make infants sick. For this reason, both the World Health Organization and the Food and Agriculture Organization of the United Nations recommend that infants at greatest risk of infection—those younger than two months old, born at a low birth weight, or born prematurely—receive liquid rather than powdered formula. Yet most hospitals routinely give mothers powdered formula samples in gift bags when their newborns are discharged.

Recently, formula companies have added probiotics, live intestinal bacteria, to their powdered infant formulas to help prevent diarrheal infections. This poses a dilemma for parents, as the instructions say to mix the powdered formula with cool water so these beneficial bacteria will not be destroyed. But the World Health Organization advises always mixing powdered formula with boiling water, to kill any dangerous bacteria that may be present in the formula.

Infant formula may contain other toxins besides bacteria. High levels of aluminum have been identified in most formulas. In 2008 some formulas were found to contain another toxic chemical as well. After Chinese manufacturers poisoned thousands of infants in China by adding melamine to formula to fake higher protein levels, the U.S. Food and Drug Administration (FDA) announced that it could not establish any safe level of melamine in formula. The FDA then tested the most popular brands of formula sold in the United States to be sure they were free of melamine. Apparently because the chemical is used in some plastic food packaging and in a cleaning solution used on food processing equipment, some of the U.S. formulas were found to have trace amounts of melamine. The agency then changed its view, and declared that the amounts of melamine found in U.S. formulas were acceptable.

From time to time, manufacturing errors in the production of infant formula have had serious consequences. More commonly, though, contaminants are introduced at home. Babies have suffered lead poisoning when their formulas have been mixed with tap water high in lead content. Water pollution is a potential problem even if water is purchased in a sealed bottle. And older feeding bottles can contain toxins that can leach into the baby's formula (see page 153).

Formula-feeding has other risks for babies:

- Formula-fed infants have higher incidences of colic, constipation, and allergic disorders. In fact, a significant number of babies are allergic to formulas, both those based on cow's milk and those based on soy.
- Formula-feeding appears to be one of several factors implicated in sudden infant death syndrome (SIDS). Babies who have received formula, in any amount, have a doubled risk of SIDS at one month of age compared with babies who are exclusively breastfed. (The reason for this is unknown. Perhaps it's that breastfed infants are generally healthier than formula-fed babies and therefore resistant to whatever causes SIDS.)
- Tooth decay, malocclusion (improper meeting of the upper and lower teeth), and distortion of the facial muscles may also directly result from sucking on bottles.

Some studies suggest that the benefits of breastfeeding extend into later childhood, adolescence, and adulthood. Breastfed babies have lower cholesterol levels and less coronary artery disease, on average, when they become adults. Breastfeeding is protective against chronic digestive disorders, such as Crohn's disease and ulcerative colitis. Although asthma rates are not significantly different between breastfed and non-breastfed babies, adults who were breastfed have a lower rate of asthma. Breastfed babies have a smaller chance of developing obesity, which can start with overfeeding in infancy, and both type 1 (juvenile-onset insulin-dependent) and type 2 (late-onset) diabetes. Cancers, including leukemia and cancer of the lymph glands, are also less common in children who were breastfed.

There is mounting evidence that artificially fed infants more often develop learning disorders and generally experience lower levels of intellectual functioning. Recent large-scale, international studies confirm previous studies' findings that children who were breastfed have higher IQs and perform better in reading, writing, mathematics, and other school subjects. Studies also reveal that it is breast milk, not the act of breastfeeding, that is responsible for this superior cognitive development.

Breastfeeding helps, of course, in establishing a close bond and meeting the emotional needs of a child. Nursing women produce hormones that promote a physiologic bonding between mother and child. And in what better way can a baby be nurtured, comforted, and made to feel secure than snuggled within his mother's loving arms, against the warmth of her breast?

Although some rationalize that bottle-feeding mothers can capture a similar warm feeding relationship, in reality they do not. This is partly because bottle-feeding doesn't require much human contact. The bottle-fed baby generally receives less stroking, caressing, and rocking than the breastfed baby. He is talked to less often, and he spends more time in his crib away from his parents. Although no one knows how prevalent the practice of propping bottles for young infants is, probably the overwhelming majority of babies who are able to hold their own bottles become almost entirely responsible for feeding themselves.

For all of these reasons, the American Academy of Pediatrics recommends that infants be offered only breast milk for the first six months after birth, and that breastfeeding continue throughout the first year and then as long as mutually desired.

WHAT'S IN IT FOR MOM?

Although the health of an infant and the emotional benefits of breastfeeding are reasons enough to nurse, women frequently have other motives. Experienced nursing mothers boast about the ease and convenience of breastfeeding. They are often quick to add that information, guidance, support, and reassurance were essential at the start. After the first few weeks, however, nursing a baby simplifies life considerably.

Nursing saves money. Feeding your baby on 8-ounce cans of ready-to-feed formula would cost about $4,000 for the first year of life. Using 32-ounce cans instead would cut the cost to about $1,800. Concentrated formula, which must be reconstituted with water, would cost about $1,500 for the year, and using powdered formula would cut the price a little more, to about $1,200.

Most experienced nursing mothers are glad not only that they don't have to buy formula but that they don't have to prepare bottles. Instead up getting up at night to fix a bottle, you can simply pull the baby to your breast and doze off again. You can go on outings with your baby without carting around formula, bottles, and nipples. (But just because the breastfed baby is easy to take along doesn't mean she can't be left behind. When you and your infant must be apart, you can leave your own milk for her. See chapter 6 for more information.) Many mothers have been grateful that they could nurse their babies through natural disasters such as storms, flooding, and fires when formula and clean feeding supplies were unavailable.

Many women worry about how they will look after they have had a baby. The fat you accumulate during pregnancy is intended for caloric reserves while nursing. Rigorous dieting is not a good idea during the nursing period, but it isn't necessary, either; most mothers find that they gradually lose weight while they are breastfeeding so long as they are not overeating. Women who formula-feed their babies may have a much harder time losing the fat they gained during pregnancy. Furthermore, two separate studies confirm that breastfeeding mothers who nursed for three months or longer after each birth had less belly fat than mothers who did not breastfeed, and no more belly fat than women who had never been pregnant.

Breastfeeding has other beneficial effects on a woman's body. Recent studies have found that women reduce their risk of type 2 diabetes by as much as 12 percent for each year they breastfeed. Swedish researchers have determined that mothers who nurse for at least 13 months cut their risk of developing rheumatoid arthritis in half. Many studies report lower rates of ovarian cancer and breast cancer among women who have breastfed, and it appears that the risk of cancer decreases the longer a woman nurses. New studies also reveal that breastfeeding has a significant impact on reducing the risk of developing heart problems in women. While it is well known that obesity, high cholesterol, and diabetes all lead to heart disease, it is less known that breastfeeding reduces the risk of all these. There is some evidence, too, that nursing offers protection against developing osteoporosis (brittle bones) later in life. And breastfeeding generally lengthens the time before menstrual periods resume after childbirth; most nursing women have no menstrual cycle for several months to two years after delivery, so long as they are nursing frequently. Recent studies comparing breastfeeding and bottle-feeding mothers suggest a lower rate of postpartum depression among nursing mothers as well.

Breastfeeding will be inconvenient. In fact, experienced nursing mothers boast about the ease and convenience of breastfeeding.

Breastfeeding will be painful. Normally, women find nursing comfortable and pleasurable. Some women develop sore nipples during the early days of nursing, but most soreness can be avoided by correctly positioning the baby at the breast (see "Positioning at the Breast," page 29). You may have heard that babies sometimes bite their mothers while nursing. When a baby is sucking, his tongue covers his lower gums and teeth so he cannot bite. Still, some babies do occasionally bite at the end of feeding, usually during a period of teething. Most babies learn very quickly not to do this.

Breastfeeding will be embarrassing. Although we all know that making milk is the natural function of our breasts, many of us feel embarrassed about exposing them. At first you may be more comfortable nursing in private, but most women find that, with a little time and experience, nursing in the presence of others can be discreet and comfortable.

Breastfeeding will tie you down. In fact, you can take your nursing baby anywhere with as little equipment as a spare diaper.

You'll have to stop breastfeeding when you go back to work. Today, a growing number of women are combining motherhood, nursing, and working, and doing it quite successfully, thanks to recent advances in milk collection and storage equipment. Having a healthy baby is especially important to a working mother, and breastfed babies are sick less often.

Breastfeeding will ruin the shape of your breasts. Pregnancy typically causes the breasts to enlarge and sometimes to develop stretch marks. During the first few months of nursing, women whose breasts are normally small or medium-sized generally find them to be bigger. As the baby gets older and begins nursing less often, most women notice their breasts reduce in size. At weaning, the breasts typically appear smaller still and somewhat droopy, but within six months they often resume their usual size and shape. A recent U.S. study found that increased maternal age, more pregnancies, higher body-mass index, larger pre-pregnancy bra size, and smoking were all independent risk factors for sagging breasts. But women who nursed generally had no more sagging than women who bottle-fed.

Your milk may be inadequate for your baby. Some mothers wonder if their diet, breast size, or temperament will keep their milk from being rich or abundant enough. None of these factors affect the amount of breast milk produced, which depends on the frequency of feedings and the baby's effectiveness at the breast. And the quality of a mother's milk is rarely an issue.

Some mothers are repelled by the smell and taste of many formula preparations, not to mention the unpleasant odor of the bowel movements and spit-up milk of the formula-fed baby and the stains formula may leave on clothing. Breast milk smells sweet, if it smells at all, and as long as a baby is exclusively breastfed, her spit-up and bowel movements smell mild and inoffensive.

BREASTFEEDING ISN'T ALWAYS EASY

If breastfeeding is natural, it must be easy, right? Sometimes it isn't. Today, close to half of all mothers who start out nursing their babies give it up within the first six weeks. The reason for this failure is rarely that the mother is unable to produce enough milk. Typically, it is because she is alone in her efforts to nurse. All too many new mothers know little about the nursing process and the breastfed infant, have little or no guidance, and lack support while they are learning. Although breastfeeding is natural, it is not instinctive—it must be learned. The chapters that follow will tell you what you need to know.

Many excellent books have already been written on the benefits of nursing over artificial feeding methods. I set out, however, to provide mothers with a practical guide for easy reference throughout the nursing period. The first part of the book provides basic information about the breast, preparation for nursing, and nursing during the first week; the remainder of the book is intended for reading as the baby and the nursing relationship grow and develop. There are chapters on each of the three later phases of nursing—from the first week through the second month, from the second month through the sixth, and after the sixth month. Following each of these chapters is a Survival Guide—a quick yet thorough reference for almost any problem you or your baby may encounter during the phase covered. Although you may rarely need to consult the Survival Guides, I have included them to ensure that, when you do, you will be able to identify and resolve your problem as quickly as possible. Because many nursing women occasionally find themselves in need of medication, Dr. Philip O. Anderson has provided an appendix on drugs and their safety for the breastfed baby in *The Nursing Mother's Companion, 7th edition* (Harvard Common Press, 2017).

Mothers who nurse do so not only because they want the very best nourishment and protection for their babies and because they personally derive many practical benefits from breastfeeding, but simply because they enjoy the experience. The loving relationship established between mother and infant at the breast is emotionally fulfilling and pleasurable. You'll know no greater reward as a mother than witnessing your child grow from your body—first in the womb, and then at the breast.

CHAPTER 1

LOOKING FORWARD:
Preparations During Pregnancy

- Learning about Breastfeeding
- Your Breasts
- Ensuring the Purest Milk

- Planning for a Normal Birth
- Planning for the First Days
- Planning for the First Weeks

YOU MAY HAVE DECIDED TO NURSE your baby long before you became pregnant. Or perhaps you have just begun to consider breastfeeding. Although nourishing a baby at the breast is natural, many new mothers are surprised to find it is a learned skill—one that usually takes several weeks to master.

Success at nursing often depends upon a woman's confidence and commitment. You can develop your confidence by learning as much as possible about breastfeeding ahead of time. You can strengthen your commitment to nurse by developing a strong support system for yourself.

LEARNING ABOUT BREASTFEEDING

Generations ago, most new mothers turned to their own mothers for support and guidance on breastfeeding. Happily, many women today can do so, too. But many can't.

If your mother didn't breastfeed, or if she gave it up quickly, there are several ways you can learn about nursing ahead of time. Reading about it is certainly beneficial. In some communities, breastfeeding classes are offered. Expectant mothers are also most welcome to attend La Leche League meetings, which are held monthly in most areas. La Leche League is the organization of nursing mothers whose purpose is to support breastfeeding worldwide. In some areas, other groups, such as the Nursing Mothers Counsel, provide classes and telephone counseling for pregnant and nursing women. In addition, hospitals, county health departments, and WIC (the Special Supplemental Nutrition Program for Women, Infants, and Children) programs may sponsor prenatal breastfeeding classes.

Another excellent way to learn about breastfeeding is to spend time with women who are nursing their babies. It may be that you have never seen, close up, a mother and baby breastfeeding. Most nursing mothers will delight in your interest, and one or two may become good sources of information and support for you in the days to come. Be sure to ask them about their first weeks of nursing. Most likely you will hear of a variety of experiences, and perhaps you will develop a sense of what the early period of breastfeeding can be like.

YOUR BREASTS

During pregnancy, many changes occur in your breasts in preparation for nourishing your baby. In early pregnancy, you probably noticed they were more full and tender than usual. Their increasing size during the first few months of pregnancy is caused by the development of the milk-making structures within them. Most women prefer to wear a supportive bra throughout pregnancy, although a few women are just as comfortable without one. From early or mid-pregnancy on, your rib cage expands. You will probably find that your bra band feels tighter, and this may require you to purchase new bras or bra extenders.

As your breasts grow in size, the blood flow to them increases, and veins in the breasts may become clearly visible. Some women develop stretch marks on their breasts, like the ones that can occur on the abdomen during pregnancy.

The nipple and the area around the nipple, the areola, may double in size and deepen in color; this darkening may serve as a visual cue to the newborn. Also during this time, small glands located in the areola, known as Montgomery's tubercles, become pronounced. Their function is to secrete an antibacterial lubricant that keeps the nipple moist and protected during pregnancy and breastfeeding. This is why soaps and special creams are unnecessary in caring for your breasts, and may even be harmful: soaps remove the breast's natural lubricant, and creams may interfere with its antibacterial action.

The nipples often become more sensitive during pregnancy. Some women find that their nipples even hurt when touched. This sensitivity diminishes as pregnancy advances; it should not make breastfeeding uncomfortable. Other women enjoy the sensitivity and feel great pleasure when their breasts are fondled during lovemaking.

By the fifth or sixth month of pregnancy, the breasts are fully capable of producing milk. Some women begin to notice drops of fluid on the nipple at this time. This fluid, known as colostrum, comes from several tiny openings in the nipple and is the food your baby will receive during the first few days after birth. Some women do not leak colostrum, but it is there in the breasts just the same.

As women, we all receive messages about our bodies and what they "ought" to look like. These messages affect our self-image, including our feelings about our breasts and how they look. You can probably remember how you felt about your breasts as they developed in early adolescence. You may have felt proud as they grew larger and you began wearing a bra. Perhaps you were embarrassed if they developed earlier or grew larger than the other girls'. You may have felt anxious if they took a long time to grow or self-conscious if they were small.

Even now you may wish that your breasts were smaller or larger, fuller or less droopy. You may not resemble the women with "perfect" breasts portrayed in photographs of nursing mothers. Women with large breasts, especially, often feel insecure about nursing, fearing that their breasts will grow much larger still or leak milk excessively. Actually, large breasts seldom grow bigger after delivery, and they tend to leak less than small breasts.

Each woman's breasts are different from all others, but most breasts, regardless of size, are perfectly designed for their ultimate purpose—to nourish and nurture our children. The breasts not only provide an infant with superb nutrients for growth and development but offer the warmth, the comfort, and the security that every growing baby needs. In this respect, they are most beautiful.

Cross-section of a lactating breast

The Making and Giving of Milk

After the birth of your baby, colostrum is readily available for her first nursings. Colostrum is the ideal food for her first days; it is both perfect nutritionally and important for protection against infection. Mature milk generally appears by the second or third day, but occasionally not until the fourth or fifth day or even later. The late onset of milk production, which is becoming a common problem, may be related to events that occur during birth (see "Planning for a Normal Birth," page 15).

A woman's body is signaled to initiate milk production with the delivery of the placenta. This causes the hormone prolactin to activate the milk-producing cells of the breast. The initial manufacture of milk occurs whether the baby nurses or not. Continued milk production is another matter. This depends on frequent and regular stimulation of the breast and the drainage of milk. The baby's sucking stimulates the nerve endings in the breast, which in turn trigger the release of the two hormones essential to milk production and release—prolactin and oxytocin.

Prolactin, as mentioned earlier, activates the milk-producing cells in the breast to manufacture milk. Oxytocin is responsible for the release of the milk from the tiny sacs where the milk is made. This release is referred to as the ejection or let-down reflex. As the baby nurses, the milk is propelled forward toward the nipple. It is the baby's job to get the milk out by compressing the areola with her tongue and gums as she nurses. During the early months of her life, your baby will receive plenty of milk as long as you nurse her frequently (at least eight times in 24 hours), she latches on and sucks properly, and you allow her a sufficient amount of time to complete each feeding. This is because breastfeeding works by supply and demand. The more your breasts are stimulated and emptied by the baby's sucking, the more milk you will produce.

ENSURING THE PUREST MILK

A mother may occasionally wonder if her milk is entirely safe for her child. Most frequently, this concern arises because she needs to take medication. Although most medications pass into the breast milk, the vast majority pass in only small amounts and are considered safe for the nursing infant. A comprehensive guide to drugs in breast milk, by Dr. Philip O. Anderson, can be found in Appendix D in *The Nursing Mother's Companion, 7th edition* (Harvard Common Press, 2017). Another source of such information is LactMed, an online database developed by Dr. Anderson for the National Library of Medicine. You can find LactMed in the list of databases at www.toxnet.nlm.nih.gov.

More and more questions have arisen about the environmental pollutants we are exposed to, such as insecticides and other toxic chemicals. Many of these substances are stored in fatty tissues of the body; as a result, small amounts may be detected in breast milk. Experts on the subject, however, have been unable to identify any risks to the baby from such amounts, and most believe that the nutritional and immunological benefits of breast milk far outweigh the possible risks of environmental pollutants. Sadly, our children receive even greater exposure to some of these chemicals in the womb than they do at the breast.

If you want to minimize your baby's exposure to toxic chemicals, follow these guidelines during pregnancy and as long as you are breastfeeding:

- Stop using pesticides in the home, in the garden, and on pets.
- Avoid exposure to organic solvents, which are in paints, furniture strippers, gasoline fumes, non-water-based glues, nail polish, and dry-cleaning fluids. Air dry-cleaned and mothballed clothes outdoors before wearing them, and avoid permanently mothproofed garments.
- Avoid eating fish species that have been found to have high levels of mercury and PCB, including shark, swordfish (also known as *kajiki*), king mackerel (which is among the species known as *saba* in Japanese restaurants), tilefish (also known as golden or white snapper), and fish caught in contaminated waters, especially the Great Lakes.

SEAFOOD, SAFE AND NOT

The U.S. Food and Drug Administration says that pregnant women should avoid eating shark, swordfish, king mackerel, and tilefish but can safely eat 12 ounces (340 grams) per week of any other types of cooked fish. The Environmental Working Group is even more conservative; this nonprofit organization suggests also avoiding fresh tuna (including varieties sold in sushi restaurants as ahi, maguro, meji, shiro, and toro), sea bass, Gulf Coast oysters, marlin (makjiki), halibut, pike, walleye, white croaker, and largemouth bass, and eating no more than 3 to 6 ounces per month of canned tuna, mahi-mahi, blue mussels, Eastern oysters, cod, pollock, Great Lakes salmon, Gulf Coast blue crab, wild channel catfish, yellowtail (known in sushi restaurants as hamachi, kanpachi, inada, or buri), bonito (katsuo), wild trout, and lake whitefish.

- Safe fish and shellfish, with mercury levels lower than 0.2 parts per million, include farmed trout, farmed catfish, fish sticks, shrimp, pollock, wild Pacific salmon, haddock, summer-caught flounder, croaker, clams, flatfish, mid-Atlantic blue crab, freshwater sport fish, and scallops. Check with your state or local health department about the safety of local species.
- Adopt a diet low in animal fat by choosing lean meats and low-fat dairy products.
- Avoid smoking and the company of those who smoke around you.
- Carefully wash or peel fresh fruit and vegetables. Avoid crash diets, which can increase the excretion of toxic substances into breast milk.
- If you work with chemicals, ask your doctor to refer you to a specialist who can advise you about their safety.

PLANNING FOR A NORMAL BIRTH

Over the past two decades, the numbers of mothers who have their labor induced, who have epidural anesthesia, and who deliver by cesarean section have skyrocketed. It is now known that these high-tech interventions often affect breastfeeding.

A complicated birth often ends with the separation of mother and baby. This may make the start of breastfeeding more difficult. All too often, a complicated birth also means the late onset of milk production. Several factors may be responsible: a long labor, epidural anesthesia, the use of synthetic oxytocin (Pitocin) to augment or induce labor, and the administration of large volumes of intravenous fluids. When milk production is delayed beyond 72 hours after birth, the newborn may become jaundiced, lose too much weight, and require supplemental feedings. A mother in this situation becomes more likely to abandon nursing.

A complicated birth often doesn't begin naturally but is induced by the breaking of the bag of waters. A doctor may suggest doing this when a mother nears or passes her due date. Induced labor all too often makes other medical interventions necessary. The rupture of the membranes may or may not stimulate labor, but it certainly increases the risk of infection to mother and baby. Once the bag of waters is broken, the clock begins ticking. In most cases, the baby needs to be delivered within 24 hours to minimize the chance of infection.

Sometimes problems during pregnancy make induction a good choice. It may be risky for the baby to remain in the uterus when pregnancy has lasted 42 weeks, when the mother has high blood pressure or an infection of the uterus, or when she has another health problem such as diabetes. Induction may also be the best option if the baby stops growing or if the amount of amniotic fluid is very low. But many doctors schedule inductions for the convenience of mothers, physicians, and hospital staff. A doctor may persuade a mother by describing induction as a routine procedure to avoid a middle-of-the-night run to the hospital and to guarantee that certain family members can be in attendance, or by voicing concern about the baby's size. Some mothers may request induction simply because they are tired of being pregnant.

None of these are good reasons for induction. Studies of thousands of cases have shown that inductions increase the incidence of labor complications and surgical delivery without improving newborn outcomes.

Nature begins preparing for birth during the last weeks of pregnancy. The baby drops down into the pelvis; the cervix tilts forward and begins to soften. The baby's lungs mature, he receives maternal antibodies that will protect him against infection in the early weeks of life, and he puts on a layer of fat. His body stores more iron, and he develops a coordinated sucking and swallowing ability. When the baby is ready to be born, he releases a small amount of a hormone that in turn stimulates the mother's body to secrete the hormones that initiate labor. When the baby, maternal hormones, uterus, cervix, and placenta are ready, labor begins. When labor begins on its own in this way, the labor tends to be easier, and the baby is usually born ready to breastfeed.

A mother who has an induction usually finds herself admitted to the hospital before labor is well established or even begun. If her due date was incorrectly estimated, the baby may be born weeks early. A developmentally immature newborn is at increased risk for complications such as temperature instability, low blood sugar, respiratory problems, and jaundice. Babies born three weeks or more early often don't learn to nurse well until near the time that they were meant to be born.

Mothers whose labors are lengthened and complicated by medical interventions tend to get their milk in later, and their babies tend to be less able at the breast. In general, a baby's breastfeeding ability is highest when the mother has given birth with neither intravenous narcotics nor an epidural. The baby's breastfeeding ability is lowest when the mother has used both intravenous and epidural drugs during labor.

Despite high satisfaction with pain relief, many mothers who have undergone epidurals report low satisfaction with their birth experiences. If you're sure you need medication in labor, you might ask for patient-controlled epidural anesthesia, or PCEA. Available in many hospitals and birth centers, PCEA allows a mother to give herself a bolus of narcotic and anesthetic when she feels the need. The dose is low, so it blocks the pain sensors but allows more movement in bed. Once the cervix is totally dilated, the epidural is turned off so the mother can respond to her desire to push. The mother's recovery tends to be better after PCEA; she can walk about sooner, and because walking may help prevent her bladder from becoming distended and may also prevent excessive bleeding. Because the baby has taken in less narcotic with PCEA, he tends to show a more normal interest in and ability at the breast.

PREPARE FOR A NORMAL BIRTH

- Attend childbirth classes, preferably ones taught by certified Lamaze or Bradley instructors, to learn more about normal birth.
- Recognize that your due date is approximate. Let your caregiver know that you prefer to wait until labor begins on its own.
- If your caregiver is concerned about the well-being of the baby, ask to have a non-stress test (electronic fetal monitoring) every two to four days for reassurance that the baby is well.
- Stay at home during early labor until your water breaks or your contractions are coming every 3 to 4 minutes and are lasting for 1 minute.
- Consider hiring a doula to assist you in coping with the discomforts of labor and birth.
- When you begin to push, try to rest between contractions. Push only when the urge comes or when your caregiver or nurse directs. Short pushes, of no more than 4 to 6 seconds each, will help conserve your energy.
- Take advantage of a water tub or shower to lessen the intensity of contractions.
- Try to delay an epidural until after labor is well established and your cervix is dilated 5 centimeters.
- If you feel you need pain medication, ask about PCEA.
- Once your cervix is completely dilated, use upright positions to assist gravity and to increase the diameter of your pelvis, so as to help the baby descend through the birth canal.
- When you begin to push, try to rest between contractions. Push only when the urge comes or when your caregiver or nurse directs. Short pushes, of no more than 4 to 6 seconds each, will help conserve your energy.

PLANNING FOR THE FIRST DAYS

Nipple Preparation

Often mothers who plan to breastfeed are advised to prepare their nipples during pregnancy. In fact, studies have shown that nipple "toughening" maneuvers, such as brisk rubbing or twisting, do little to prevent soreness during early breastfeeding. Whether or not they have especially sensitive skin, blondes and redheads do not generally experience any more nipple soreness than other women. Sore nipples are usually prevented by correct attachment of the baby at the breast (see "Positioning at the Breast," page 29).

If you have had one or both nipples pierced, remove the jewelry before giving birth and leave it out as long as your baby is nursing. You'll probably be able to nurse without complication, but you may find that you leak milk from the site of the piercing.

One preparation is very important during pregnancy: You should make sure your nipples can extend outward. Your baby may have difficulty grasping the breast if the nipples do not protrude enough on their own or cannot be made to protrude. Even if you had a breast exam earlier in your pregnancy, your nipples may not have been fully checked. Take the time to perform your own assessment.

First, look at both your nipples. They may protrude, or one or both may be flat, dimpled, folded in the center, or inverted. Next, do the "pinch test": Gently squeeze just behind the nipple with your thumb and forefinger. This imitates the motion your baby will make while nursing. See how both nipples respond. If your nipples are flat, pull them outward to determine if they can lift away from the inner mass of the breast. The chart below will help you determine whether you need to take further steps to minimize initial nursing difficulties.

When nipples need correction. The flat nipple that cannot be pinched outward, or the nipple that moves inward or flattens when compressed, is said to be "tied" to the inner breast tissue by tiny adhesions. The physical changes of pregnancy help the nipples to stand out, but one or both may still need correction. In this case, special plastic breast shells may solve the problem before breastfeeding begins.

USUAL NIPPLE APPEARANCE	APPEARANCE WHEN PINCHED	
	SATISFACTORY	NEEDS CORRECTION
Protruding	Nipple stays protruded	
Flat	Nipple can be pinched outward	Nipple moves winward or cannot be pinched outward
Dimpled or folded	Entire nipple extends outward	Nipple moves inward or flattens
Inverted	Entire nipple extends outward	Nipple extends out only slightly, remains inverted, or inverts further

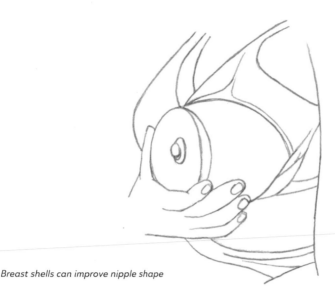

Breast shells can improve nipple shape

Worn inside the bra, breast shells exert a steady but gentle pressure on the areola and cause the nipple to extend outward through the opening in the shell. This may help to loosen adhesions beneath the nipple. Breast shells should be worn as soon as you have determined that improvement is needed, ideally from about mid-pregnancy on. They can be purchased in most maternity shops or ordered through Medela. Gradually work up to wearing the shells most of the day, letting comfort be your guide.

The Postpartum Setting

Too few mothers realize ahead of time the tremendous effect the immediate postpartum experience—in a hospital, in a birth center, or at home—can have on their breastfeeding success. It is most worthwhile to evaluate the situation you will be in after delivery to make any necessary arrangements for early nursing.

The maternity unit's policies should encourage mothers and babies to remain together for the first few hours after birth, or at least assure that nursing takes place within the first two hours, when the baby is likely to be alert and eager to suck. Ideally, the baby isn't swaddled, weighed, bathed, and placed in a crib after birth but simply dried and placed naked against his mother's bare chest; then they are both covered. Newborns treated this way tend to have more respiratory stability and higher blood-sugar levels and cry much less than other babies. If the birth was unmedicated, the baby will generally be quiet but alert and able to crawl to the breast and latch on unaided in 30 to 60 minutes (you can see a video of a newborn crawling to the breast at www.breastcrawl.org). Weighing, bathing, eye treatment, and other baby care procedures are best postponed until after the first feeding.

> Studies show that mothers who nurse during the first two hours after giving birth are much more likely to be successfully nursing weeks and months later.

Breastfeeding goes best when nursing is frequent, every one to three hours, during both day and night. "Rooming in" with the baby, at least during the day and evening, is conducive to frequent nursing and allows the mother and baby to become better acquainted before going home. Preferably, the nursing staff does not routinely give the babies water or formula supplements, as this lessens their interest in nursing and sometimes interferes with their ability to breastfeed. It can be an added bonus if the nurses enjoy assisting breastfeeding mothers or if one nurse is specifically responsible for breastfeeding counseling.

Some women have the opportunity to select among several hospitals or birth centers for their delivery. If you are making such a choice, be sure to get a recommendation from your childbirth educator or a local breastfeeding counselor. She will probably know which places are most supportive of nursing mothers and infants. Even if only one hospital is available to you—and many birth attendants practice at only one—it is well worth your time to ask about the policies of the maternity unit. This will help ensure that your nursing gets off to the best possible start.

Take advantage of the maternity tours, teas, and classes that most hospitals and birth centers offer, or call the postpartum unit to learn about policies and routines. Be sure to inquire:

- How soon after delivery will I be able to nurse? What if I have a cesarean birth?
- Will I be able to hold the baby skin-to-skin right after the birth?
- How often is nursing encouraged during the day and at night?
- Can the baby stay in the room with me? If not, how often and for how long will we be together?
- What assistance with breastfeeding does the nursing staff offer?
- Does the staff avoid supplemental bottle-feeding?
- Is there a lactation professional on staff?

In 1990, the United Nations Children's Fund and the World Health Organization created an award of recognition for those hospitals worldwide that have enacted ten policies to support breastfeeding mothers and babies. Hospitals that have implemented the "Ten Steps" are awarded the designation "Baby-Friendly." As of this writing, 203 U.S. hospitals and birthing centers in 45 states and the District of Columbia are considered baby-friendly, while another 500 are working toward the designation. When inquiring about a hospital's breastfeeding policies, ask if it has earned or applied for the Baby-Friendly certificate. If it has, you can be assured that the nurses are committed to your breastfeeding success. If it hasn't, perhaps your inquiry will inspire the hospital to enact baby-friendly policies. You can find all "Baby-Friendly" hospitals in the United States listed at www.babyfriendlyusa.org.

If the nurse is friendly and receptive to your questions, you might also ask which pediatricians she feels are particularly knowledgeable about breastfeeding and supportive of it.

If you are planning an early discharge from a hospital or birth center, or will be delivering at home, you may also want to inquire about home visits by a nurse, lactation professional, or midwife during the first few days.

The Baby's Doctor

Your breastfeeding experience can be greatly influenced by your choice of physician for your child. You may want a pediatrician for your baby, or you may prefer to use a family practitioner, perhaps the one who may attend your baby's birth. In selecting a doctor, start by getting the names of some who are said to have a positive attitude about breastfeeding. Ask your obstetrician, midwife, childbirth educator, or a lactation professional for recommendations. You might also inquire about physicians in your area who work with nurse practitioners. These nurses have advanced education and training in well-baby care, and they usually provide mothers with extra attention and counseling on a variety of parental concerns, including breastfeeding.

Most doctors and nurse practitioners will set aside time for a preliminary visit with expectant parents. Usually this visit is free of charge. Be sure to visit at least two before making a final decision, even if the first one seems satisfactory. At each office, meet the nurse. She will often be the one who will answer your questions or concerns when you call during office hours. She can be a good resource for you, especially if she has breastfed successfully herself or has a special interest in breastfeeding.

Let the doctor or nurse practitioner know that you are going to breastfeed your baby. To gauge his or her overall support of nursing mothers, ask what the recommendations would be should you experience difficulty in breastfeeding. The best pediatric practitioners offer practical assistance with breastfeeding or referrals to lactation professionals. Other practitioners provide reassuring words about feeding infant formula. Take time to discuss your preferences for feeding the baby in the hospital. If the maternity unit's policies are not ideal, ask about written orders to allow early nursing and rooming-in and to prevent the feeding of supplements to your baby. A few pediatric practices have lactation consultants on their staff or can refer you to experienced lactation consultants in your area. There may be other questions you will want to ask about the hospital or birth center, or about well-baby care. Bring a list with you so you don't forget any of them. Be sure to inquire about any necessary procedures for notifying the doctor or nurse practitioner when the baby is born. It is often said that the pediatrician takes care of the parents perhaps even more than the child. Trust your intuition when making your final choice about which pediatrician, family doctor, or nurse practitioner is right for you.

Nursing Bras and Pads

During the early weeks of breastfeeding, the average breast weighs three to four times as much as it did before pregnancy. Although a bra isn't an absolute necessity in this period, you'll probably be more comfortable in one, at least if it fits well. If you leak milk and want

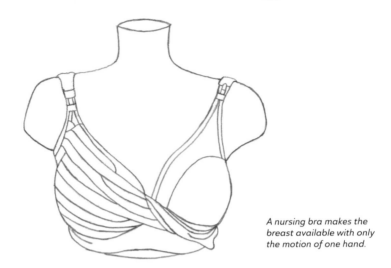

A nursing bra makes the breast available with only the motion of one hand.

to use breast pads, you'll definitely need a bra to hold them in place. A stretch bra that can be pulled out of the way may work fine if you're small-breasted, but otherwise you may prefer a nursing bra with removable cup flaps.

After you give birth, both your cup size and band size will most likely change. If you buy a nursing bra in early pregnancy, it may not fit when milk production begins. A better time to shop for nursing bras is during the last couple of weeks of pregnancy or after your baby is born. To be on the safe side, limit your purchase to two or three bras; you'll be more sure of the size and style that suits you after a few weeks of nursing.

The salesperson in the maternity shop or department may be able to help you choose a bra that will fit well while you are nursing. If she doesn't know a lot about bras, though, you can figure out your size yourself by following these guidelines: While standing, wearing an unpadded bra and breathing normally, measure your chest just under your arms with a tape measure. Round up to an even number of inches; this number is your band size. Now measure around your body at the fullest part of your bust. As shown in the chart on page 23, the difference between the bust measurement and band size determines your cup size.

Since finding larger bra sizes can be difficult, you may have to use a mail-order supplier. To check a bra for fit, fasten it on the outside row of hooks. Before raising the straps over your shoulders, bend forward, allowing your breasts to fill the cups. Now stand straight, and adjust the straps.

Check the cup fit. When the flaps of a nursing bra are hooked at their highest points, the cups should have just a little extra room at the top for when milk production begins. If the cups are roomier than this, try a smaller cup size. If your breasts are overflowing at the top, outsides, or center, you need a larger cup size.

Next check the bottom band. While fastened on the outside row of hooks, the band should be snug; an inner row of hooks will allow you to tighten the band as your rib cage contracts after birth. Check to see that the band is level all around or slightly lower in the back. If the bra rides up in the back, the shoulder straps may be too tight. Otherwise, try a larger cup size.

Aside from a good fit, other valuable features of a bra for breastfeeding include all-cotton or microfiber cups to absorb moisture, nonelastic straps for better support, and front-flap fasteners that are manageable with one hand.

A word about underwire bras: Poorly fitted ones are associated with plugged milk ducts and breast infections. If you want to wear an underwire bra while nursing, it is very important to get one that fits properly. The bend of the wire must be wide enough to fall where there are no milk ducts—that is, well behind the breast tissue. If you have a lot of breast tissue below the armpits, as many women do, a soft-cup bra is definitely preferable. If you do use an underwire bra while nursing, alternate it with a soft-cup bra, and never wear the underwire bra during sleep.

You may also wish to purchase breast pads before delivery, to keep your bra and clothing dry during the early weeks of nursing (not all women leak, so you may want to start with just one pack). Breast pads are sold in two varieties, disposable and reusable. Whichever you select, be sure the pads do not contain plastic or waterproof liners, as these can contribute to nipple soreness. If you prefer, you can use handkerchiefs or cut-up cloth diapers instead of commercially made pads.

Sometimes mothers consider using plastic breast shells instead of pads to keep dry. The primary purpose of these shells is to improve nipple shape. When they are routinely worn in place of pads, milk may leak excessively.

DIFFERENCE BETWEEN BUST MEASUREMENT AND BAND SIZE	CUP SIZE
Up to 1 inch	A
1 to 2 inches	B
2 to 3 inches	C
3 to 4 inches	D
4 to 5 inches	DD or E
5 to 6 inches	F
6 to 7 inches	G
7 to 8 inches	H

A comfortable armchair can make positioning your newborn at the breast much easier and provide more support for you while nursing. An upholstered living-room, dining-room, or office chair with arms, or a wooden rocking chair, may make a great place for nursing your baby. If your breasts are large, a recliner may be most comfortable. Consider borrowing an appropriate chair or buying one secondhand if you can't afford a new one.

You can get by without an armchair, of course. Most couches are too deep to sit up straight on, and propping yourself upright against the headboard of your bed makes it hard to position the baby and may contribute to poor posture and muscle fatigue. But either a couch or bed can work well if you lean far back and position your baby for latch-on using "biological nurturing," as described in chapter 2.

> Babies need to spend most of their time in a horizontal position, whether in someone's arms or on a safe, level surface. A bouncer seat, bassinet, or blanket on the floor is a better place than a plastic carrier to leave your baby for extended periods. Or carry your baby in a pouch or sling, keeping your arms free for other things. Holding, rocking, and carrying your baby against your body will stimulate his physical and mental development while strengthening the loving bond between you.

Although ordinary bed pillows can work well in helping to position a baby for nursing, a variety of pillows are marketed specifically for this purpose, and they are becoming very popular for the early weeks of nursing. If you'd like to try one of these pillows, choose one with flat surfaces rather than one that is shaped like a croissant. The latter type creates a gap between the pillow and the mother's body, and the baby tends to slip down in between.

Many mothers have found that a footstool specially designed for nursing is very helpful in reducing the strain of holding the baby at the breast. The angled stool raises the mother's feet and legs, lifting her lap. This relaxes her abdomen and supports her lower back, preventing arm and shoulder strain.

Some mothers buy breast pumps before delivery. Although a pump is not a necessity for everyone, you may at some time want to use one. Or you may prefer to learn the technique of hand expression, which is described on page 136. Your insurance provider may be required to provide you with a breast pump, although the models that they offer may not be very effective, so check carefully. Be sure to ask about the window of time you have for ordering your pump. *The Nursing Mother's Companion*, 7th ed. (see "Suggested Supplemental Reading," page 182) has detailed information on working with your insurance carrier to obtain a pump. You might also speak with a lactation consultant, who will have experience with high-quality breast pumps and may even have them available for sale if your insurance carrier does not offer breastfeeding equipment to nursing mothers. Many mothers end up disappointed with pumps they buy at discount, baby, and big-box stores.

Some mothers need a clinical-grade electric pump in the first few days after delivery. Whether you buy another sort of pump or not, find out where you can rent a clinical-grade pump should the need arise. If your baby isn't nursing well upon leaving the hospital or is at risk of underfeeding for another reason (see page 39), you should go home with a clinical-grade electric pump, ideally with a double collection kit.

In the first weeks after giving birth, many mothers find it helpful to keep a log of their nursings and their babies' stools and urine output. One study has suggested that women who keep such logs tend to breastfeed longer than those who don't. You might consider purchasing *The Nursing Mother's Companion Breastfeeding Diary* (see "Suggested Supplemental Reading," page 182) as a handy record book and keepsake for the early weeks.

PLANNING FOR THE FIRST FEW WEEKS

During your first few weeks of motherhood, caring for the baby and yourself will take just about all of your time and energy. Most new mothers find they are often tired and have emotional highs and lows. Planning ahead can make these important first weeks go much more smoothly for both you and your family.

If your partner can possibly manage to take time off from work, by all means encourage him to do so. Not only can he help in fixing meals, managing the household, and caring for any other children at home, but he also needs and deserves time to get to know the baby. And he can be a great source of support and encouragement while you are learning to breastfeed.

Other family members can also make these weeks easier, but invite them to stay with you only if you feel they will make a positive contribution and be supportive of your nursing.

Perhaps some of your friends in the area have already offered to help when the baby arrives. There are many things they can do, like fixing a meal, washing a load or two of laundry, running errands, minding any older children, or spending an hour or so straightening up your house.

It's also a good idea to stock up on groceries before the birth. Include foods that are easy to prepare and plenty of things to drink. You may also want to plan some simple menus or freeze a few dinners ahead of time.

About half of American women who start out breastfeeding give up and begin bottle-feeding within the first three months after birth. As Dana Raphael wrote more than thirty-five years ago, "The odds in our culture today are stacked heavily against successful breastfeeding, and the emotional price for failure is high." Although more breastfeeding help is available now, those words still hold true. Mothers frequently give up breastfeeding in the learning stage because they have too little information, guidance, and support. When a nursing mother is encouraged and cared for by others, her motivation can carry her through almost any difficult situation. When she feels alone and unsupported, however, the nursing relationship seems to fall apart at the slightest provocation.

As enthusiastic as you may feel now, you probably have difficulty imagining that during the early weeks you may sometimes doubt your ability to nurse. In fact, many new mothers experience periods of anxiety while they are learning to breastfeed. If you are lucky, you can turn to your own mother for advice and reassurance about nursing.

Many of today's grandmothers, however, nursed for only a few weeks. You may hear them say, "The baby was never able to take the breast" or "I just didn't make enough milk" or "Nursing hurt too much." Comments such as these reflect an era when women received little encouragement and support in their efforts to nurse, and the lactation consulting profession was in its infancy. Consider for a moment the idea of giving birth all alone. Awful, right? It is probably important to you that someone you love and trust will be with you, encouraging you each step of the way. During your early weeks of breastfeeding you need the same kind of support—the presence of someone who provides reassurance, guidance, and encouragement.

You may be fortunate enough to have friends who have nursed—or are nursing—their babies, and a partner who believes with you that breastfeeding is healthy and natural. Even so, you may discover in time that not everyone in your life shares your feelings about breastfeeding. In fact, many people feel indifferent, and some downright opposed, to this way of feeding and nurturing a baby. Your partner, mother, or best friend may not be entirely enthusiastic about your decision. Some people may even try to discourage you along the way. Perhaps they feel a bit threatened, fearful, or even jealous of the intimate relationship you will be establishing with the baby. The sad fact of the matter is that despite the renewed enthusiasm of young women today toward breastfeeding, many new mothers still get too little support —from family, friends, health professionals, and society in general.

> You can find the names of International Board Certified Lactation Consultants in your area by going to www.ILCA.org and clicking on "Find a Lactation Consultant."

Develop a support system for yourself ahead of time. Let your partner and other family members know how much breastfeeding means to you and how important they will be to your success. If they have concerns or fears about nursing, find out what they are and provide them with the information they need to correct any misconceptions. If you have older children, talk with them about nursing so they know what to expect.

Be sure to identify sources of guidance. Perhaps you are close to women who have successfully nursed their babies. Many WIC (the Special Supplemental Nutrition Program for Women, Infants, and Children) offices provide breastfeeding support and guidance. Take time to find the names of lactation professionals in your community. Your childbirth educator, your hospital's maternity unit, or your obstetrician's or pediatrician's nurse may know of some. In addition, your insurance carrier may be required under the Affordable Care Act to cover the cost of consulting a lactation professional with no cost sharing. When you have gathered these supports, you will have stacked the odds in your favor.

CHAPTER 2

OFF TO A GOOD START:
The First Week

- In the Beginning
- Ensuring Your Milk Supply
- The First Week of Nursing

YOU MIGHT EXPECT THAT AFTER THE WORK of labor and birth a mother and her newborn infant would be too exhausted to greet each other. But no matter how fatigued birth may have left her, the mother usually brightens with renewed energy to explore her baby. Some mothers seem to meet their infants for the first time with puzzlement, as if searching for some sign of familiarity. Others react as if they have always known this tiny being and are overjoyed to meet him at long last.

After several minutes of adjustment to breathing, the temperature change, and lights and sounds, the unmedicated infant likewise becomes alert, opening his eyes and moving his mouth. The newborn who is placed skin-to-skin with his mother is soon crawling toward the breast and is actively rooting about. With his fists to his mouth, or perhaps his lips against his father's arm, he seeks out the comfort of the breast. Ideally, the mother and baby should be left skin-to-skin until the first nursing takes place.

IN THE BEGINNING

Colostrum

Throughout the first two hours after birth, the infant is usually alert and eager to suck. At this time he is most ready for his first nursing.

It is not unusual to hear a first-time mother tell a nurse, "I don't think I have anything yet to feed the baby." Although small in amount, colostrum is available in the breast in quantities close to the stomach capacity of the newborn. This "liquid gold," which is often yellow but may be colorless, is more like blood than milk in that it contains protective white blood cells capable of attacking harmful bacteria. Colostrum also acts to "seal" the inside of the baby's intestines, preventing the invasion of bacteria, and provides the baby with high levels of antibodies from the mother. Not only does colostrum thus offer protection from sickness, it is also the ideal food for the newborn's first few days of life. It is high in protein and low in sugar and fat, making it easy to digest. Colostrum is also beneficial in stimulating the baby's early bowel movements. The black, tarry first stools, called meconium, contain bilirubin, the substance that causes newborn jaundice. Colostrum in frequent doses helps eliminate bilirubin from the body and may lessen the incidence and severity of jaundice.

In the hospital the first nursing may take place in the delivery room, the birthing room, or the recovery area. With minimal assistance from your nurse or partner, the baby will probably seek out your breasts and suck within the first hour or so. It is ideal for the baby to be naked against your bare chest.

Many specialists believe that when the first nursing is delayed much beyond the first two hours, the infant may be somewhat reluctant to take the breast thereafter. Most babies fall asleep about two hours after birth, and they become more difficult to rouse over the next few hours. Nursing without delay also boosts the confidence of the mother and stimulates the action of hormones that cause the uterus to contract and remain firm after delivery. These contractions may help speed delivery of the placenta and minimize blood loss afterward (breastfeeding alone is insufficient, however, in the case of postpartum hemorrhage, when prompt intervention by the medical staff is essential). During the first few days after birth, some mothers feel these contractions, or "afterpains," while nursing. Mothers who have had other children may be quite uncomfortable with afterpains. If you experience these contractions during breastfeeding, you can ask for a mild pain reliever like acetaminophen (Tylenol) or ibuprofen (Motrin, Advil) an hour or so before nursing.

Should you not have the opportunity to nurse right after delivery, or if you can't persuade your baby to take the breast, don't get discouraged. Many mothers have established successful nursing hours or even days after giving birth.

Just the Breast

When you have finished your first nursing in the hospital, let the nurses know (if you have not done so previously) that you prefer your baby be given no supplementary bottles of water or formula and no pacifiers. Water or formula is unnecessary, and artificial nipples may cause your baby to have difficulty recognizing your nipple while she is learning to breastfeed. A recent study reveals that mothers whose babies received supplements or pacifiers in the hospital were far less likely to achieve exclusive breastfeeding.

Newborns do not normally require any fluids other than colostrum (the exception is the baby who has low blood sugar—because her mother is diabetic, her birth weight was low, or she underwent unusual stress during labor or delivery). Supplemental feedings, moreover, can be harmful: They may cause the baby to lose interest in the breast and to nurse less frequently than needed. This is because bottle nipples may lessen the baby's instinctive efforts to open her mouth wide, as she needs to do to grasp the breast, and condition her to wait to suck until she feels the firm bottle nipple in her mouth. The baby who has sucked on bottle nipples may also become frustrated while nursing, because milk does not flow as rapidly from the breast as it does from the bottle.

Giving newborns large amounts of water can be dangerous. Because young babies can't excrete water quickly, large amounts can lower sodium levels in their bodies, causing complications that include low body temperature and, sometimes, seizures.

A newborn trained to take a pacifier may fail to recognize her mother's soft, short nipple and therefore have trouble latching on to the breast. Introducing a pacifier now could lead to later problems, too. Recent studies associate the use of pacifiers with early weaning, and older babies who use pacifiers are more likely than others to have frequent ear infections.

Some hospitals now have policies against giving bottles and pacifiers to nursing newborns, but not all do. To be sure all the nurses know of your preference, ask them to place a sign on the baby's crib like this one:

TO ALL MY NURSES:

While I'm here and learning to breastfeed, PLEASE, NO BOTTLES OR PACIFIERS. My mom will be happy to nurse me whenever I fuss.

Thanks!! Baby Reynolds

Time at the Breast

Many doctors and nurses tell mothers that to prevent sore nipples they should limit their nursing time during the first several days. Probably nothing else about breastfeeding is as poorly understood as the causes of sore nipples. It may be explained that keeping feedings short will prevent soreness and will help "toughen" the nipples. Actually, sore nipples usually result from improper positioning of the baby on the breast, not from long nursings. Another myth often heard by new mothers is that the breast "empties" in a prescribed number of minutes. Most newborns require 10 to 40 minutes to complete a feeding. As long as your positioning is correct and nursing is comfortable, there is no need to restrict your nursing time. Besides being unnecessary, limiting nursing time may frustrate the baby and lead to increased engorgement when milk production begins.

Positioning at the Breast

A baby is correctly positioned at the breast when he has latched on to it with a wide-open mouth so that his lower gum is well below the base of the nipple on the areola, the dark area around the nipples. In this off-center or "asymmetrical" position he will compress the sinuses located beneath the areola to draw out milk. If he instead latches on to the nipple only, or latches on with the nipple centered in his mouth, and starts sucking, the nipple will probably become sore and cracked and may even bleed. The baby will also be unable to compress the sinuses beneath the areola well and may therefore get too little milk.

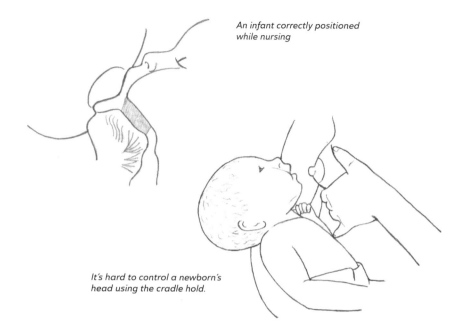

An infant correctly positioned while nursing

It's hard to control a newborn's head using the cradle hold.

Probably the most important skill for you to master, initially, is that of getting the baby on the breast correctly. Some mothers can do this easily, but many need practice.

Cradle (or cuddle) hold. This hold, in which the baby's head is held in the crook of the mother's arm, is considered the classic breastfeeding position. I have come to believe that for most new mothers and babies, this position is neither the easiest nor the most effective for getting a baby well latched on to the breast. In the first few weeks after birth, a baby hasn't developed enough muscular coordination of the head and neck to easily latch on without help; she needs a good deal of direction from her mother. But it is difficult to direct a newborn's head accurately with the inside of one's forearm. Also, it is usually not possible to get an off-center latch using this position. Although most mothers sooner or later begin using the cradle hold for most of their daytime nursings, in the early days of breastfeeding the crossover and football holds are generally more useful.

Crossover hold. Take time to position yourself comfortably. If you are nursing in a hospital bed, sit up as straight as possible with a pillow behind you. As soon as you are able, sit in a chair with arms (most couches are too deep). Unwrap your baby; this will encourage his interest in latching on and make it easier for you to check his position. Place one or two pillows on your lap so that the baby is at the level of your breast. Lay him on his side with his chest and abdomen against your body.

Instead of placing the baby's head in the bend of your elbow, as in the cradle hold, hold him with the opposite arm so that your hand rests between his shoulder blades and supports the back of his neck and head. Place your thumb behind and below one ear and your other fingers behind and below the other ear. Tip his head back slightly so that when you pull him onto the breast, his chin will reach it first. Now shift the baby, if necessary, so that the area just above the upper lip—not his mouth—is right in front of your nipple. In this position he is most likely to latch on asymmetrically, with his lower jaw far below the base of the nipple.

If you're starting on the left breast, hold it with your left hand so that your thumb is positioned at the margin of the areola, about 1½ inches from the nipple, at the spot where the baby's upper lip will touch the breast (or at about two o'clock, if you imagine a clock face printed on your breast). Place your index finger the same distance from the nipple at the spot where the baby's chin will touch the breast (or at about eight o'clock). Gently compress the breast to match the shape of your baby's open mouth.

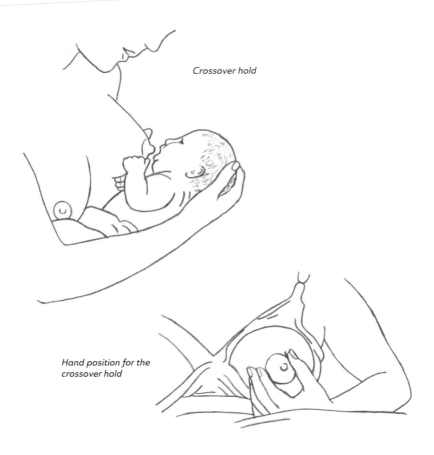

Crossover hold

Hand position for the crossover hold

Before you bring the baby onto the breast, you must stimulate him to "root." With the baby's forehead tipped back, touch the baby just under the nose with your nipple, and wait until he opens his mouth wide. When his lower jaw is dropped all the way down, quickly bring his shoulders and head together to the breast. With his head tipped slightly back, his chin should reach the breast first. Don't lean into the baby or move your breast. Keep the areola compressed until he begins sucking. You'll know that he is well latched on if his lips are far apart and flared, if he has more of the bottom of the areola in his mouth than the top, and if you feel comfortable.

You may need to repeat this process a few times before the baby latches on correctly. Common mistakes include lining up the baby's mouth rather than the upper lip area with the nipple, pulling the baby on before his mouth is wide open, not pulling him on quickly enough or far enough, and letting go of the breast before he is well latched on.

When you're first learning to get a baby latched on, it helps to see someone else do it. There are many wonderful videos about breastfeeding. Dr. Jane Morton, a pediatrician in general practice, a clinical professor at Stanford University, an executive board member of the American Academy of Pediatrics' Section on Breastfeeding, and a fellow of the American Academy of Breastfeeding Medicine, has produced wonderful videos about breastfeeding. "A Perfect Latch" is intended for physicians but is also helpful for mothers who are learning to get a baby latched on. This video is available for viewing online at http://newborns.stanford.edu/Breastfeeding/FifteenMinuteHelper.html.

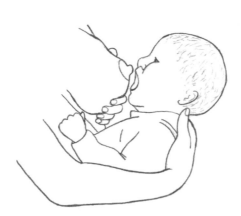

Just before latch-on: Tip the baby's head back a bit, and aim your nipple at his upper lip

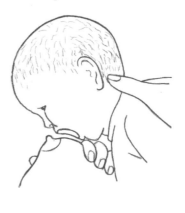

Just before latch-on, from your point of view

Once the baby is actively nursing, you'll probably need to support the breast for him by gently pressing your fingers against the underside. If your breasts are small, though, you may be able to let go of the breast or even switch arms and continue nursing using the cradle hold.

Football hold. The football hold is a great position to use in the following circumstances:

- You have had a cesarean birth and want to avoid placing the baby against your abdomen.
- You need more visibility while getting the baby to latch on.
- Your breasts are large.
- You are nursing a small baby, especially if he is premature.
- You are nursing twins.

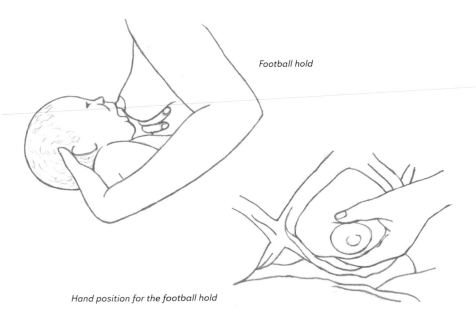

Football hold

Hand position for the football hold

Sit in a comfortable armchair with a pillow at your side to help support your arm and lift the baby. Support the baby in a semi-sitting position facing you, with her bottom at the back of the chair. Your arm closest to your baby should support her back, with your hand holding her neck and head. Place your thumb behind and below one ear and your other fingers behind the other ear. Position the baby with her head just below the breast and her nose in front of the nipple. This way she'll latch on to the areola off-center, with her lower jaw well below the base of the nipple.

Support your breast with your free hand so that your thumb is about 1½ inches above the nipple, at twelve o'clock, and your index finger is the same distance below the nipple, at six o'clock. Compress the areola with your thumb and index finger so that your hand forms a C-shape. This will more closely match your breast to the shape of your baby's mouth she can take in more of the breast. As with the crossover hold, stimulate the baby to open her mouth wide, and bring her up onto the breast.

Side-lying position. The side-lying position is an especially good choice for nursing in these cases:

- You must lie flat after a cesarean birth.
- You are uncomfortable sitting up.

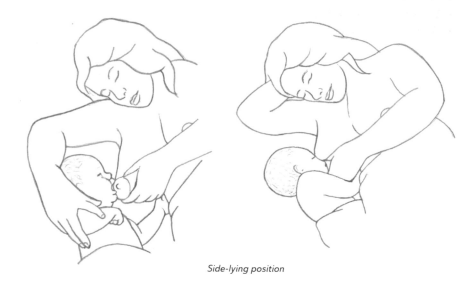

Side-lying position

- You need help from someone else to get the baby latched on.
- The baby is sleepy and reluctant to begin nursing or stay awake very long.
- You are nursing during the night.

You and your baby lie on your sides, tummy to tummy as with the cuddle hold. Place your fingers beneath the breast and lift upward, wait for the baby to root with a wide-open mouth, and then pull him in close.

The side-lying position becomes much easier after four to six weeks, when the baby has better head control and can come onto the breast without much assistance.

Biological Nurturing

Recently, a new approach to getting a newborn latched on to the breast has been described by Dr. Suzanne Colson, a nurse-midwife from England. "Biological nurturing" employs the normal reflexes of newborn infants, which Dr. Colson teaches are present in part to assist the baby to latch on to the breast by himself. The technique uses a very comfortable position for mothers and may be especially helpful with newborns who are struggling to achieve a good latch.

With this technique, the mother leans back against pillows, and the baby is placed vertically or obliquely on top of her. The baby, wearing no more than a diaper, lies against the mother's bare skin with his face on top of her breast and his feet touching her thighs so he can use his crawling reflex to reach the nipple area. The feel and smell of the breast stimulate the baby to open his mouth very wide and bob his head up and down and from side to side as he searches for the nipple. Because the mother is leaning back, the baby is able to use gravity to his advantage and so takes the nipple deeply into his mouth. The mother can support the baby's bottom with one hand and help present the breast with the other. On his website (www.breastfeedinginc.ca), Canadian pediatrician Dr. Jack Newman offers a video of a baby latching on, for the first time, with this technique—click on "Videos/Info Sheets" and then choose "Baby-Led Mother-Guided Started Upright Left Breast, Latches." To learn more about biological nurturing, visit Dr. Colson's website, www.biologicalnurturing.com.

Ending the Feeding

Waiting until your baby lets go of the nipple is the ideal way to end a feeding. If the baby does not come off the breast by himself after 20 to 25 minutes on a side, and you want to switch breasts or rest awhile, you can take him off by first breaking the suction. Even if he is not actively sucking, his hold on the nipple is tremendously strong. To release the suction, place your finger at the corner of the baby's mouth, pulling the skin gently toward his ear, until you hear or feel the release.

After taking the baby off the breast, leave your bra flaps down so that the air can dry your nipples. If your nipples are tender or damaged and you want to soothe them, you may be offered a modified lanolin preparation or a gel pad. However, recent studies suggest that using gel pads may lead to higher rates of breast infections when used by nursing mothers. If your nipples are tender or injured and you are using a nipple ointment, be sure to wash your hands frequently and especially right before nursing. I also suggest some other products for treating tender or injured nipples in "Survival Guide: The First Week," page 47.

AFTER A CESAREAN BIRTH

If you are awake for your delivery, let the staff and the baby's physician know that you wish to nurse as soon as possible. While some hospitals allow the mother to hold the baby against her skin in the operating room while she is being sutured, many do not, and, frankly, some mothers do not feel well enough to enjoy this experience. Also, surgical suites are kept cool for the doctors' comfort, and the low room temperature can cause a mother's body temperature to drop so low that she may not be able to keep the baby warm enough.

As long as neither you nor the baby is having difficulties, however, there is no reason to delay nursing for long. One option is to have a nurse or your partner bring your baby to you in the recovery room. If you were not fully conscious during the delivery, or if the doctor orders that the baby be kept in the nursery, you can still begin nursing after your initial separation.

When the baby arrives, place him against your skin, and cover him. Enjoy his attempts to crawl to the breast and nurse. If he doesn't latch on even with your help, have your partner or the nurse help you feed him in the side-lying position. Leave the side rails of the bed up so that turning will be easier. A pillow behind your back and one between your legs may be helpful.

Because you will be recovering from surgery, you will face some discomfort and possibly some difficulty in maneuvering the baby to your breast. The pain medication you'll receive, probably a narcotic, is important for your comfort during the first few days, and it will not hurt the baby. If you take the medication right after you nurse, moreover, only a minimal amount will be in your milk at the next feeding. After the first couple of days, a nonnarcotic pain reliever, like acetaminophen (Tylenol) or ibuprofen (Motrin, Advil), may be adequate to control your pain most of the time.

When you begin sitting up to nurse, a pillow or two on your lap will make you more comfortable. The football hold may work well if you want to keep the baby off your abdomen, but some mothers may not get a good off-centered latch and may find that they get sore nipples using this hold.

After a couple of days you may want to keep the baby in the room with you. Remember to ask for help whenever you need it. Sometimes the staff may forget you gave birth by cesarean.

Whether or not your cesarean was planned, your milk should come in just as if you had delivered vaginally, although it may be delayed if you had a long or complicated labor and received large amounts of intravenous fluids (see page 48).

ENSURING YOUR MILK SUPPLY

Frequent Nursing

Most babies nurse infrequently during the first 24 hours of life. But thereafter your baby should be nursing often, at least eight times in 24 hours. Studies show that the numbers of daily nursings on the second, third, and fourth days of life are directly related to how much milk is produced on days 5 and 14. Until your milk comes in, your baby needs frequent feedings of colostrum. After your milk comes in, probably about 72 hours after the birth, a good feeding every few hours will help ensure a plentiful milk supply.

During the first few days after birth, many babies are sleepy. If your newborn has not nursed after three hours (counted from the start of the last feeding), unwrap her from her blankets. Rub her back and talk to her, or place her, dressed in only her diaper, against your bare chest. She will probably then become interested in nursing.

In the hospital, keeping the baby with you in your room helps ensure frequent nursing. If you are not sharing a room with your baby, ask the nurses to bring her to you at least every three hours (more often if she fusses), including whenever she wakens in the night.

Encourage the baby to have a good feeding each time you nurse her. Until your milk is in, you can probably persuade her to take both breasts at each feeding. Listen for the sound of your baby swallowing; when you hear it, you will know that she is taking colostrum or milk.

Dr. Jack Newman, of the Newman Breastfeeding Clinic and Institute in Canada, has produced some excellent videos that show both babies who are latched on and swallowing well and others who are taking very little milk. You can find links to these videos at www.breastfeedinginc.ca. The clip entitled "Really Good Drinking" shows a baby who is a few days old. The mother's milk has come in, and the baby is vigorously sucking and swallowing. Not only can you see the baby drinking and occasionally hear him swallowing milk, but you can see that he has taken the breast deeply into his wide-open mouth. (Before the milk has come in, a baby may not swallow as much.) For contrast, you can see a baby who is only nibbling at the breast, with little if any swallowing, in the video clip entitled "Nibbling."

In the video entitled "Baby 28 Hours Old, Baby-Led Mother-Guided Latching," a lactation consultant and Dr. Newman show a mother how to compress her breast to stimulate milk flow to the baby. With the help of breast compression, this one-day-old baby begins swallowing colostrum. Breast compression is easy to do: When the baby is sucking but is not swallowing, gently squeeze the breast until the baby begins taking long sucks with pauses for swallowing.

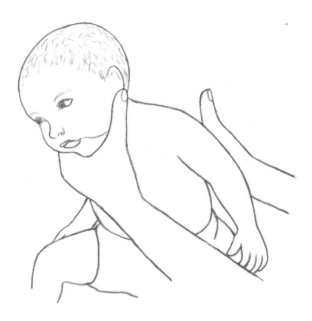

You can burp the baby by sitting her up, one hand under her jaw. Firmly pat her lower back with the other hand.

When your baby has released the nipple, or when you have nursed her for 20 to 25 minutes and she is no longer swallowing, burp her. Hold her up over your shoulder and pat her back, or sit her upright, bent slightly forward with your hand supporting her lower jaw, and firmly pat her lower back. After burping, she will probably regain interest in nursing and take the second breast. If she doesn't burp within a few minutes, just switch sides. If she refuses to nurse on the second breast or nurses for only a short time, be sure to start her on that side at the next feeding.

The first days of milk production are the critical period for determining whether a mother ends up with a generous milk supply or an inadequate one. If little milk is removed from the breast, the resulting pressure causes the breast to slow down production. If no milk is removed, milk production stops entirely (this is how women who don't nurse stop producing milk). So ensuring a good milk supply depends on having a vigorous nursing baby, or an effective breast pump, that drains at least one breast every few hours around the clock.

Avoiding Supplementals

Another way to help ensure your milk supply is to avoid supplemental feedings. Some babies develop a strong preference for an artificial nipple when a bottle is introduced during the first few days (see "Just the Breast," page 28). Glucose (sugar) water offers few calories and may discourage the baby's interest in nursing. Also, babies fed glucose water more frequently develop jaundice in the first few days after birth. After taking formula, a baby frequently will not want to nurse for four hours or longer, since formula takes longer to digest than breast milk. The decrease in breast stimulation may decrease milk production.

Putting Your Fears to Rest

In the early days of breastfeeding, you may be surprised at how often your baby wants to nurse. He may be especially fussy on the second night following birth, before milk production begins; most babies want to nurse nearly hourly during this period. Even after your milk comes in, your newborn may seem fussy and hungry much of the time. This may make you wonder if you have enough milk, and if you should pump your milk and feed it by bottle to see how much the baby is getting. Well-meaning friends and family members may even suggest you supplement your milk with formula.

Most newborns want to nurse 8 to 12 times in each 24-hour period after the first day or two of life. This frequent nursing is normal; it seldom reflects a poor milk supply, and it never reflects "weak milk." Unless you or your baby falls into one of the categories described under "Babies Who May Not Get Enough" (see page 39), your baby is probably getting plenty of milk.

Without introducing a bottle, though, how can you know your baby is getting enough? You can look for these signs of adequate milk intake:

- Your milk has come in by the third day after birth. When milk production begins, the breasts become firmer and heavier. The firmness may be less apparent with large breasts, but the breasts should still feel heavier.
- Your baby is nursing at least eight times in a 24-hour period after the first 24 hours. This means your baby is nursing every two to three hours (measured from the start of one feeding to the start of the next) during the day, with a sleep stretch of up to five hours at night. If your baby isn't nursing this often, you may have to wake her for feedings.
- Your baby is nursing for 10 to 45 minutes at each feeding and seems content after feedings. Babies vary in the length of time they nurse, but they typically need 10 to 45 minutes to complete a feeding. Although babies don't always fall asleep after nursing, they should usually seem satisfied after feedings.
- Your baby has several periods of swallowing during each feeding. When babies are getting milk, they take long, drawing sucks and can be heard swallowing or gulping (see page 41).
- Your breasts feel softer or lighter after the baby has nursed. Once milk production has begun, you should be able to feel a decrease in fullness or heaviness after feeding your baby.
- Your baby is having bowel movements every day, and by the fifth day they have turned yellow. This is the clearest sign that a baby is getting enough colostrum at first, and then later enough breast milk. Most newborns have at least two to three bowel movements each day during the first month. Only after the first month is it normal for breastfed babies to go several days without a bowel movement.
- Your baby is wetting more diapers by the fifth day after birth. Before your milk comes in, your baby will urinate infrequently, but by the fifth day you should notice more frequent and wetter diapers. Be aware that most disposable diapers today are so absorbent that they can make wetness difficult to detect.

If not all of the points just listed hold true for you and your baby, you should have him weighed and examined. In the first four to five days after birth, a baby loses weight. After the fifth day, a baby should gain an ounce every day. An initial loss of 10 percent or more of a baby's birth weight suggests the baby is underfed. Even if your baby has lost less than 10 percent of his birth weight, have him weighed again in a couple of days to see if he has started gaining an ounce per day.

Babies Who May Not Get Enough

Some mothers and babies at risk for underfeeding can be identified even before the milk comes in. This group includes:

- Babies who are born at 37 weeks' gestation or earlier (see "The Near-Term Baby," page 79)

- Babies weighing less than 6 pounds at birth (see "The Near-Term Baby," page 79)
- Babies who may have poor muscle tone, such as those with Down syndrome (see "Developmental and Neurological Problems," page 89)
- Babies who have unusual conformations in their mouths, such as a short frenulum (the string of tissue on the underside of the tongue) near the tongue's tip, a high palate (see page 66), or a cleft lip or palate (see "The Baby Who Has Not Yet Nursed," page 66, and "Cleft Lip and Palate," page 88)
- Babies who aren't yet latching on or sustaining sucking 24 hours after birth (see "Sucking Problems," page 69)
- Mothers with nipples as large as or larger in diameter than a quarter (see "Sucking Problems," page 69)
- Mothers who have very soft breasts with no noticeable change in fullness and no other signs of milk production at 72 hours following birth (see "Late Onset of Milk Production," page 48)
- Mothers who have had previous breast surgery involving an incision around the nipple or areola, such as in some breast augmentation and reduction procedures
- Mothers who have polycystic ovary syndrome, or PCOS
- Mothers who have widely spaced, long, thin breasts that did not get larger in pregnancy and that may differ markedly from each other in size
- Mothers who have placental fragments still in their uterus (see "Late Onset of Milk Production," page 48)

If you or your baby falls into one of these risk groups, a few days of sluggish nursing and limited milk removal could have a devastating effect on your milk production, even if breastfeeding seems to be getting off to a good start. Consider renting a clinical-grade breast pump, preferably with a double collection kit, which may be more reliable than your baby in stimulating continued milk production. Starting on the third day after birth, pump for 5 to 10 minutes with a double collection kit right after each daytime and evening nursing. If you don't have a double collection kit, pump each side twice, for a total pumping time of 10 to 15 minutes. If your baby isn't able to latch on or clearly isn't sucking effectively, start pumping earlier than the third day, and pump for 10 to 20 minutes with a double collection kit or 10 to 15 minutes per side without one. This should ensure that you'll have an abundant milk supply even if your baby's sucking is sluggish. You can freeze the pumped milk for later use.

If your baby is latching on and sucking, watch her closely for the reassuring signs of adequate milk intake listed on page 39. Weigh her at three to four days of age and approximately every two days thereafter until she is clearly gaining an ounce a day. If she loses 10 percent or more of her birth weight or does not gain an ounce a day after five days of age, she needs your pumped breast milk or formula as a supplement. If she has regained her birth weight, you can gradually stop pumping over a few days. Before returning the pump, though, make sure the baby has gained an ounce a day since the last weighing. See "Treatment Measures for Underfeeding," page 73.

THE FIRST WEEK OF NURSING

Although most unmedicated babies are alert and eager to nurse during the first two hours after birth, during the next few days they may sleep much of the time. The average baby, after the first couple of days, begins to wake up to nurse about every one to three hours. At night, he will sleep from one to five hours at a stretch. If your baby is not waking on his own to nurse at least eight times in each 24-hour period, including at least once in the night, wake him for feedings.

The typical length of a feeding varies greatly from baby to baby. A baby who is "all business"—who sucks and swallows with few pauses—may complete a feeding in as little as 10 minutes. At the other extreme is the baby who sucks and swallows five or six times and then pauses. This pattern of frequent pausing may extend a feeding beyond 40 minutes. Most babies' feedings fall between these extremes; the average is 20 to 30 minutes. Although your baby may not fall asleep after feeding, he should seem content.

A baby who takes longer than 45 minutes to complete most of his feedings may not be getting sufficient amounts of milk and should be weighed to make sure that he has not lost too much weight or, after the fifth day of life, that he is gaining weight.

After your milk comes in, you should hear a lot of swallowing while nursing the baby. Swallowing sounds something like "eh, eh, eh." Some babies gulp noisily, whereas others swallow more quietly. Between swallows, babies take long, drawing sucks. (They take short, choppy sucks when they are not swallowing milk.) These long, drawing sucks usually occur in bursts, that is, five to ten continuous sucks followed by a resting pause. Babies who are taking enough milk usually have several bursts of continuous sucking and swallowing during a feeding.

You should not hear clicking noises while your baby nurses. Clicking often means that the baby is not sucking adequately and therefore may not be receiving enough milk. Some babies make clicking sounds if they have a very high palate (roof of the mouth). The baby may not be able to press the nipple up against it if it is very high, deeper than the underside of a teaspoon. Some babies have such high palates that you will need to place your cheek on their chest to be able to see the top of it. The baby should have such a strong hold on the breast that the nipple does not easily slip from his mouth when you pull him slightly away. His cheeks should remain smooth with each suck; dimples on the cheek while nursing are a sign of inadequate suction and faulty sucking (see "Sucking Problems," page 69, if your baby's cheeks are dimpling or if you don't hear much swallowing). One exception to clicking being abnormal can occur when a baby is getting so much milk and is swallowing so much that she momentarily unlatches without coming off the breast, which also causes a clicking sound.

During the first day after birth, babies sometimes spit up mucus they have swallowed during delivery. Occasionally a baby will gag on this mucus. After the first 24 hours, this is usually no longer a problem.

Some babies also spit up colostrum or milk. The amounts are usually smaller than they seem, though you may wonder if your baby is keeping anything down. Spitting up a teaspoon or two after feedings is normal for some babies in the first week.

Babies also get hiccups, often after a feeding. Hiccups are the result of the baby's full tummy. You may remember the baby hiccuping in utero after drinking amniotic fluid. If the baby starts hiccuping after nursing at the first breast, it may be difficult to interest him in the other. You don't need to give him water or anything else. The hiccups are painless for him; just wait until they go away.

The baby's first stools, called meconium, are black and sticky. Having bowel movements every day and yellow stools by the fifth day usually indicates an adequate intake of colostrum, first, and then breast milk. Frequent yellow stools are one of the surest signs that a newborn is getting enough to eat. Most newborns have at least two bowel movements each day during the first month.

The yellow stools of a breastfed baby are soft, loose, or even watery, and sometimes they look seedy. Babies normally strain and grunt when passing their stools. This does not mean they are constipated.

Wet diapers are usually infrequent in the first few days, but they should be more frequent and wetter by the fifth day. Eight or more diapers wet with pale urine each day, along with daily yellow stools, are usually a sign of sufficient milk intake. (This rule may not hold true if the baby is receiving water or formula supplements.)

All newborns lose weight after birth. Expect your baby to lose 5 to 9 percent of his birth weight. He should begin gaining weight by the fifth day, about an ounce a day.

Caring for Your Breasts

Your daily bath or shower is sufficient for cleaning your breasts. Avoid getting soap or shampoo on the nipple and areola; this would counteract the naturally occurring oils that cleanse this area. Antiseptic applications to the nipples are also unnecessary, but do take care to wash your hands before nursing.

You will probably want to wear a nursing bra for convenience and comfort, especially after your milk comes in. Again, bras with cotton or microfiber rather than synthetic cups allow for better air circulation to the nipples.

If the baby does not come off the breast by herself when the nursing session is over, take care to release the suction by pulling with your finger at the corner of the baby's mouth, toward her ear. Leave your breasts exposed to the air for 5 to 10 minutes before covering up.

In the past, nursing mothers were discouraged from using nipple creams, because some women develop sore nipples in reaction to preparations containing lanolin, vitamin E, or cocoa butter. Some lanolin preparations were also discovered to be contaminated with pesticide residues. However, a purified form of lanolin has been developed; it rarely causes allergic reactions. Another aid for sore nipples are gel pads, but while they are soothing to sore nipples, they have been associated with breast infections. Other options for soothing tender or injured nipples are discussed in "Survival Guide: The First Week," page 47.

If you are using plastic breast shells to improve the shape of your nipples, you may find during the first few weeks that they cause your milk to leak excessively and keep your nipples damp. You might try placing the shells in your bra just 10 to 20 minutes before the feeding (milk collected this way should be discarded if it has been in the cups longer than a half hour or so). Don't routinely use breast shells in place of nursing pads; this usually causes more leakage. Breast shells should be washed after each nursing in hot soapy water and rinsed thoroughly.

When Your Mature Milk Comes In

Mature milk production generally begins on the second or third day after birth, but occasionally not until the fourth day or later (if your milk hasn't come in by the third day, see "Late Onset of Milk Production," page 48). At first the milk will be mixed with colostrum, and so will be pale orange in color. After a few days the milk will become whiter. This mature milk will look more watery than cow's milk; it may resemble skim milk.

Most women notice that their breasts become larger, fuller, and more tender as the mature milk comes in. Large-breasted women may notice only a change in heaviness. This change, known as engorgement, is caused by increased blood flow to the breasts as well as beginning milk production. Fullness may be more apparent if your breasts are normally small or medium-sized. They may feel lumpy, and the lumpiness may extend all the way to your armpits, since milk glands are also located there. After nursing, your breasts should feel softer or lighter.

Engorgement normally lasts 24 to 72 hours. During this time a nursing bra will provide support and comfort. Frequent nursing, at least every two to three hours, is the best treatment. Heat treatments such as warm showers, hot packs, and heating pads may worsen the swelling. You may get relief, though, with cool applications to the breast and by gentle massaging or compressing the breast while the baby is nursing. This will encourage more milk to let down. It is important to pay careful attention to the way the baby latches on while the breast is engorged. When latch-on is incorrect, because the baby isn't positioned well or the areola is overly full, soreness often follows. If the areola is hard, you can express some milk, by hand or with a pump. (For further advice on managing engorgement, see "Engorged Breasts," page 47.) When you put your baby to breast, you may feel any of these normal sensations: warmth, relaxation, sleepiness, thirst, and even hunger.

It is normal for milk to leak from the breasts. When the baby nurses at one breast, milk may drip or even spray from the other. This leaking may continue for several weeks, or it may never happen at all. For women who leak milk, nursing pads are usually necessary to prevent wet or spotted clothing. You can buy the pads in two varieties: reusable and disposable. A new type that helps lessen leaking is called LilyPadz. Made of gas-permeable silicone, these pads apply a gentle pressure on the nipple to stop milk leakage.

FROM HOSPITAL TO HOME

In many hospitals, it is customary at the time of discharge to give new mothers an array of sample products that manufacturers would like them to try. You might conclude that the staff endorses these products, but this is not necessarily so. One of the gifts is usually something that may be labeled a "breastfeeding kit"—infant formula (often powdered, although powdered formula isn't safe for newborns—see page 5), bottle nipples, and a pamphlet on breastfeeding, which may contain misleading information. Since you have chosen to breastfeed, it is best to leave the kit behind. You won't be needing it.

Well worth taking home, however, are the names and telephone numbers of people who have a good reputation for helping nursing mothers and infants. Ask any nurse who has been encouraging or helpful with your early breastfeeding for this information. She may know of volunteers in La Leche League or the Nursing Mothers Counsel, or experienced lactation professionals in your community.

When you're getting ready to leave the hospital by car, have ready some small blankets to support your baby in her car seat, even if you'll have a short drive home. Because a newborn can't control her head well, she needs special support to allow her to breathe freely while riding in a car seat. A study of car seat models (Tonkin et al., 2006) found that all newborns need blanket rolls at either side of the body and another across the top of the head. Many also require a blanket roll between the crotch belt and the legs to keep from sliding down in the seat. This is particularly important for infants born early. The Snuggin Go infant positioner is a soft insert that helps preterm and term infants stay well positioned in their car seat.

If a baby has been born before 37 weeks' gestation, the American Academy of Pediatrics recommends that the hospital staff observe her while she reclines in a car seat to be sure her breathing, heart rate, and oxygen levels remain normal. Nurseries that care mainly for full-term babies may not be aware of this recommendation, so you may need to ask for your baby to be monitored before she is discharged.

At home. As any experienced nursing mother can tell you, the first few days at home with a baby are exhausting and, at times, emotional. These days are best spent caring for only yourself and the baby. Besides recovering from the birth, you are doing the important work of getting to know your baby and learning to breastfeed. Rest and a quiet, pleasant environment are important in preventing anxiety and "baby blues." Try to eat well, but don't worry if your appetite has lessened; this can be normal during the first couple of weeks after delivery. Do be sure to drink enough water in order to stay hydrated. Ideally, you should spend the first several days nursing and resting with the baby, while a supportive partner or helper (or both) manages your home, meals, and callers.

If you have another child or children, you'll want help with them, too. Otherwise you may find yourself feeling suddenly, unexpectedly impatient or irritable with a beloved older child. When my second child was born, I found myself wishing someone could take away my nine-year-old for a while. Such feelings may arise from a natural protective urge that allows a mother to focus her total attention on the vulnerable newborn; shifting hormones and lack of sleep may contribute, too. Other species also defend their babies aggressively. For instance, picking up the new babies of a household pet may make the new mama growl, though in a few weeks she may not care at all when someone handles them.

Because all newborns are susceptible to declining oxygen levels when they remain seated for a long time, researchers recommend minimizing car travel and avoiding the use of car seats as carriers and other seating devices, such as swings, in the early months of life.

In women, as in cats and dogs, such feelings usually lessen over time. In the meantime, they present a fine opportunity for your older child to strengthen a relationship with Dad, Grandma or Grandpa, or another adult. This is also a great chance for your older child to learn patience and responsibility. You can encourage him to accept the big-kid role by saying outright that "the baby comes first." Your child may feel proud to help by fetching a diaper or glass of water, and he may later be able to apply the baby-comes-first principle with other helpless creatures, such as pets.

Some parents find it helpful to keep a log of the baby's feedings and urine and stool output during the early days of breastfeeding. This information may reassure them that the feedings are going well and help a doctor or lactation professional analyze any problem that may arise. If you don't have a copy of The Nursing Mother's Companion Breastfeeding Diary (see "Suggested Supplemental Reading," page 182), your caregiver may give you a blank log, you can find one on the Internet (for example, at www.kellymom. com), or you can create your own. For each 24-hour period, include the number of nursings, the number and color of stools, and, perhaps, the number of wet diapers. There is seldom any reason to keep such a log after the baby has regained his birth weight, which usually happens between 10 and 14 days of age. There are also now smartphone apps to keep track of infant feedings.

Regardless of how you gave birth, you may continue to require pain medication for the first week or so at home. Use over-the-counter pain relievers such as acetaminophen (Tylenol) or ibuprofen (Motrin, Advil) as often as you need for afterpains or pain from an episiotomy or cesarean incision. Use narcotic pain relievers only when the over-the-counter medications are not enough.

Taking narcotic pain relievers often and for more than one week after birth can, in some instances, make a baby sleepy and in rare cases lead mothers to experience withdrawal symptoms when the medication is stopped. Withdrawal symptoms may include depression, anxiety, crying, difficulty sleeping, nausea, vomiting, diarrhea, excessive sweating, and dilated pupils. Some of these symptoms mimic a normal postpartum emotional upset, but others do not.

It is not uncommon for things to suddenly "fall apart" shortly after a new mother comes home from the hospital. Suddenly responsible for a new baby, you may feel shaky, and at times your confidence may vanish. The dramatic hormonal shift that begins immediately after birth may also affect your emotional state for a while. You may find yourself exhausted and upset—especially if you've been taking responsibility for more than the baby and yourself.

Many new mothers have times when they feel that nursing "isn't working" and think about giving it up. Combined with the mood swings that follow birth, fears that the baby may not be getting enough milk, struggles with getting the baby to latch on, or problems like sore nipples, nursing can be overwhelming. A partner may become very concerned when they witness these struggles and emotional episodes, and he may become anxious to find a solution. If your partner can't "fix" your breastfeeding problems, they may encourage you to give up on nursing.

Your partner will be more supportive if he feels he plays an important role in helping the family adjust after childbirth. So encourage him to help—even if he puts the diaper on backward! He might hold the baby while you nap, put meals together, tidy the house, care for other children, and even track down a lactation consultant for you.

Despite tearful moments, rest assured that most early nursing difficulties can be overcome with patience and help. Don't hesitate to seek assistance. Just a phone conversation with a knowledgeable person may be enough to get you and your baby back on track.

The postpartum period is a time of physical and emotional adjustment. As with most of life's great transitions, this one is usually accompanied by some turmoil. It will take several weeks, and most of your time and energy, to get to know your baby and learn how to care for her. So don't do more than you must, and accept offers for help. Adjusting to motherhood is always easier when you are supported and cared for by others.

The First Week

CONCERNS ABOUT YOURSELF

- Engorged Breasts
- Late Onset of Milk Production
- Sore Nipples
- Breast Pain
- Leaking Milk
- Let-Down Difficulty
- Milk Appearance
- Difficult Latch-on: Flat, Dimpled, or Inverted Nipples
- Fatigue and Depression

CONCERNS ABOUT THE BABY

- Sleepy Baby
- Bowel Movements
- Jaundice
- Difficult Latch-on: Refusal to Nurse
- Sucking Problems
- Fussiness and Excessive Night Waking
- Underfeeding and Weight Loss

CONCERNS ABOUT YOURSELF

Engorged Breasts

Two to three days after a woman gives birth, her breasts usually become engorged, or temporarily swollen. The breasts typically feel fuller, although large-breasted women may notice only more heaviness. Engorgement is caused by the increased flow of blood to the breasts and the start of milk production. For some women the breasts become only slightly full, but for others they feel very swollen, tender, throbbing, and lumpy. Sometimes the swelling extends all the way to the armpit.

Engorgement may cause the nipples to flatten, making it difficult for the baby to latch on. The problem usually lessens within 24 to 72 hours, but the swelling and discomfort may worsen if nursing is too brief or infrequent or if the baby sucks ineffectively. If engorgement is unrelieved by nursing or pumping, milk production declines and ultimately stops altogether.

Although many health-care providers recommend applying direct heat (warm washcloths, heating pads, hot water bottles, or hot showers) to engorged breasts, this may actually aggravate engorgement.

TREATMENT MEASURES FOR ENGORGED BREASTS

1. Wear a supportive nursing bra, even during the night. Be sure your bra is not too tight.

2. Nurse frequently, every one and a half to three hours. This may mean waking the baby (see "Sleepy Baby," page 61).

3. Avoid having the baby latch on when the areola is very firm. To help keep the baby's mouth from sliding down onto the nipple and injuring it, use a technique by Jean Cotterman (2004): Just before nursing, soften the areola by placing two or three fingers at the base of the nipple and pressing firmly against the areola. Hold this position for at least 1 minute, and then move your fingers to a different spot at the base of the nipple and repeat the pressure. Or soften the areola and extend the nipple by manually expressing or pumping a little milk (see page 136). Wearing plastic breast shells for half an hour before nursing may also help to soften the areola.

4. Encourage the baby to nurse for at least 10 minutes or longer. It is preferable to nurse on just one side until the breast is soft, even if the baby goes to sleep, than to limit the baby's nursing time on the first side so you can nurse from both sides in one feeding.

5. Gently massage or compress the breast by squeezing it gently as the baby nurses. This will encourage the milk to flow and will help relieve some of the tightness and discomfort you feel (see page 37).

6. To relieve the pain and swelling, apply a cold pack to the breast for a short period after nursing. You can use ice in a plastic bag or, better, soak a disposable diaper in water, shape it, and then freeze it. Lay a thin cloth over your breast before applying the cold pack or diaper.

7. If you need to, take a mild pain reliever such as acetaminophen (Tylenol) or ibuprofen (Motrin, Advil).

8. If, 48 hours after your milk has come in, you still find yourself overly full right after nursing, use a pump to drain both breasts as completely as possible. In this first week, habitual pumping along with nursing can lead to more engorgement and chronic overproduction, but pumping after nursing once every 24 hours or so should relieve your engorgement, not prolong it.

9. If the baby is not nursing well enough to soften at least one breast every few hours, use a clinical-grade pump as necessary (see page 140).

Late Onset of Milk Production

Occasionally milk production is delayed beyond 72 hours; sometimes it begins days later. In the meantime, the breasts remain soft, and the baby sucks but gets little milk. In these circumstances, some babies seem sleepy and content, but most act dissatisfied. They may spend a long time sucking at the breast only to act hungry when they stop. They have infrequent bowel movements, many become jaundiced, and they lose more weight than normally expected.

Events during labor and birth can delay the onset of milk production. Overhydration with intravenous fluids during labor is a frequent cause of delayed milk production. Retained placental fragments are another possible, although uncommon, cause. It is thought that the hormones secreted by even small placental parts still attached to the uterine wall can keep the milk from coming in. Suspect retained placental fragments if you experienced postpartum hemorrhage or if, since the birth, you've had some of these symptoms: cramping, heavy bleeding, passing of tissue, foul-smelling lochia, and fever. Even some women who have delivered by cesarean have had retained placental fragments. When a doctor removes the fragments, milk production usually begins.

Most newborns lose weight following birth. While some professionals believe that a weight loss of up to 8 percent is normal, others are comfortable with a weight loss of up to 10 percent. Losing 10 percent or more of birth weight may be a red flag that the baby has lost too much weight, which can lead to dehydration, jaundice, and poor feeding.

If your milk is late coming in, you may need to supplement with whatever colostrum you can express and/or formula until it does. But you should continue to nurse frequently in the meantime.

TREATMENT MEASURES FOR LATE-ONSET MILK PRODUCTION

1. If, 72 hours after the birth, you suspect that your milk is not in, have your baby weighed. If he has lost 10 percent or more of his birth weight, nurse frequently, every two to two and a half hours during the day or evening, or more often if the baby seems hungry, and every three hours in the night, or more often if the baby wakes sooner.
2. Check the baby's weight every day or two.
3. Seek advice from a lactation professional, if possible.
4. While the baby is at the breast, listen for swallowing. When he drifts off to sleep and is no longer swallowing, massage or compress your breast (see page 37). You can also switch breasts as the swallowing slows, to help the baby wake and begin swallowing again. Massaging, compressing, and switching back and forth for 20 to 30 minutes will help stimulate the breast and maximize the amount that the baby takes.

   After each nursing, hand express your colostrum or breast milk and/or use a clinical-grade electric breast pump with a double collection kit (see page 140). You can read more about manual expression and pumping in chapter 5. You can also learn the technique of hand expression from a lactation consultant or by viewing a helpful video made by Dr. Jane Morton, Stanford University, at http://newborns.stanford.edu/Breastfeeding/HandExpression.html.

   Express or pump your breasts for 5 to 10 minutes, and then feed your baby the colostrum you collect along with any necessary formula (see Appendix). If you want to avoid using a bottle, you can offer your colostrum or milk using a spoon. Some mothers may be given or sold a supplementer by a lactation consultant for feeding the baby additional milk with a small tube while the baby nurses at the breast.

5. Consider using herbs known to stimulate milk production (see below).

6. If you have possible symptoms of retained placenta (see page 49), call your doctor or midwife.

7. When your milk comes in, refer to "Underfeeding and Weight Loss," page 73, for guidance in estimating your production and weaning your baby off expressed milk or formula. Have the baby weighed often as you gradually stop using formula and pumping. After the fifth day of life, all babies should be gaining an ounce per day.

HERBS FOR MORE MILK

Various herbs are known to stimulate milk production. One of the most effective may be fenugreek. You can make a tea from the seeds, but more convenient and effective is the capsule form, available in most health-food stores. Mothers who take three 580- or 610-milligram capsules three times a day typically notice an increase in the milk supply within one to three days. Although fenugreek capsules are usually taken for just a few days, some mothers continue to use them for weeks or months without any difficulties.

Fenugreek is generally harmless, although your sweat and urine will probably take on a distinct odor of maple. Rarely, mothers taking fenugreek report having diarrhea, but it quickly subsides when the fenugreek is stopped. There have also been reports of asthmatic women developing symptoms while taking fenugreek.

Blessed thistle (*Cnicus benedictus*) is also helpful in stimulating milk production. Like fenugreek, this herb is available in most health-food stores in capsule form. The typical dosage is three 390-milligram capsules three times a day. Consider using fenugreek and blessed thistle together to stimulate greater milk production.

Two other herbal preparations I recommend are More Milk Plus and More Milk Special Blend, both manufactured by Motherlove Herbal Company. More Milk Plus contains fenugreek, blessed thistle, nettle, and fennel, and is designed to increase milk production quickly. More Milk Special Blend, with the same herbs plus goat's rue, is designed to stimulate the development of breast tissue as well as increase the milk supply in women who have polycystic ovary syndrome (PCOS), who have a history of breast surgery involving an incision around the areola, or who have underdeveloped breasts. It is often used by mothers who are adopting. Both preparations are offered in capsule and tincture form. Tinctures are stronger and faster acting than capsules.

Another herbal preparation is Go-Lacta. Go-Lacta is made from the leaves of the Malunggay tree and has been shown to increase milk production in one study. It can be taken with other herbal supplements, like More Milk Plus or More Milk Special Blend.

Sore Nipples

There is no doubt about it: Sore nipples can make a trial of what ought to be a joyous experience. For a few days after giving birth, you may feel slight tenderness during the first minute of nursing, when the baby latches on and the nipple stretches into her mouth. Such tenderness is normal at this time.

If your nipples become really sore, however, they are probably injured or irritated and require treatment beyond simple comfort measures. It is important for you to identify the cause of the problem so that you can help your nipples heal. At any time that you are unable to tolerate the pain and the position changes recommended do not help, consult a lactation professional. If none is available, you may want to temporarily stop nursing; pump your milk with a clinical-grade rental pump using a double collection kit for 24 to 72 hours, or until the nipples heal (see page 136 for information on expressing milk).

There are two basic types of sore nipples: the traumatized nipple and the irritated nipple. The traumatized nipple may be blistered, scabbed, or cracked. The irritated nipple is very pink and often burns. Occasionally a mother may have both types of soreness at once.

In addition to the specific treatments listed for each category of sore nipples, the tips below will help speed healing and provide comfort.

GENERAL COMFORT MEASURES FOR SORE NIPPLES

1. A half hour before nursing, take acetaminophen (Tylenol), ibuprofen (Motrin, Advil), or a pain reliever prescribed by your doctor.
2. Avoid nipple shields (see page 58) for nursing, unless you are under the care of a lactation consultant. These thin, soft silicone nipple covers are designed to help infants who are having difficulty latching on to the breast. Nipple shields can make the soreness worse, and they can decrease your milk supply. Nipple shields come in different sizes; a wrong fit may not allow adequate breast compression and can cause the baby to get too little milk.
3. Do not delay nursings. Shorter, more frequent nursings (every one and a half to two hours) are easier on the nipples than longer, infrequent nursings.
4. While nursing, massage or compress your breasts (see page 37) to encourage the milk to flow and to speed emptying.
5. If you are sore during the entire feeding, restrict nursing to one breast only or restrict the time to 10 to 15 minutes per side. This will probably mean nursing more often, every hour or two. If nursing is still too painful, rent a clinical-grade pump with a double collection kit.
6. Release the baby's suction carefully (see page 42) before removing him from the breast.
7. After nursing, wash your hands and then apply a thin coating of modified lanolin (see page 42) or other ointment to your nipples to soothe them and promote healing.
8. Another soothing ointment is Motherlove Nipple Cream, which contains three herbal remedies for healing sore or injured nipples. Medical-grade Manuka honey is well known for its healing and antibacterial properties.
9. Between nursings, you might wear vented, hard plastic breast shells to keep your bra off your sensitive nipples. If you use plastic breast shells, wash them daily.
10. Avoid wearing hydrogel dressings. These cool, soothing pads may feel good but are associated with the development of breast infection.
11. Change disposable or cloth nursing pads after each nursing and when they become wet.

12. Wear cotton or microfiber bras. Other fabrics do not allow adequate air circulation.
13. Suds and rinse your nipples in your daily shower and rinse them in warm water after each nursing. Take care to wash your hands before handling your breasts.
14. If you are using a breast pump instead of nursing during a period of soreness, pump your milk often—at least eight times a day—to keep up your supply. Again, anything other than a clinical-grade rental pump with a double collection kit may not be effective enough to maintain your milk supply. (See page 136 for more information on expressing milk.)

Traumatized Nipples. Cracks, blisters, and abrasions usually result because a baby is improperly positioned for nursing; her gums close on the nipple instead of the areola. This often occurs when a baby fails to open her mouth wide enough or when her gums slide off the areola onto the nipple, commonly because the breast is engorged or unsupported. Babies who have a faulty suck or who are "tongue-tied" (see page 66) can also cause cracks, blisters, and abrasions. Cracking may also occur with irritated nipples (see page 53) and thrush nipples (see page 53).

TREATMENT MEASURES FOR TRAUMATIZED NIPPLES

1. Carefully review "Positioning at the Breast," page 00, so that you clearly understand the details of correct latch-on technique. The crossover or football hold is highly recommended. Review the video recommended on page 00. You might also try "biological nurturing" (see page 34).
2. If your breast is so full that the areola cannot be easily compressed, soften it by pressing with your finger, as described on page 00, or by manually expressing or pumping a little milk. This will allow the baby to get more of the areola into her mouth and help stimulate the milk to let down.
3. If your baby is reluctant to open her mouth wide, don't let her chew her way onto the breast. Patiently wait until she opens her mouth wide. Letting the baby suck on your finger for a few seconds may stimulate her sucking reflex and encourage her to open wider.
4. Do not hesitate to take the baby off the breast as soon as you realize that she is not in the right position. You may need to help her latch on a couple of times before you succeed at getting her far enough onto the breast. Ask your partner or a lactation consultant to observe your latch-on technique. A helper can also guide your arm when the baby opens wide so that she is pulled in as quickly and as close as possible.
5. Don't turn to a nipple shield when dealing with traumatized nipples. You may not find the correct size shield, which can make nipple pain worse or may not allow the baby to empty the breast well.
6. Apply a thin coating of modified lanolin (see page 42) or Motherlove Nipple Cream with clean hands right after nursings.

7. Consider trying medical-grade Manuka honey, which has been irradiated to destroy any botulism spores and therefore is safe to use while nursing a newborn. This honey protects against the damage caused by bacteria and has anti-inflammatory properties that can quickly reduce pain and inflammation. You can use a nursing pad to keep your nipple from sticking to your bra.

8. Ask your midwife or physician about trying APNO (all-purpose nipple ointment), Dr. Jack Newman's ointment recipe for healing sore nipples. It was developed to treat nipple soreness or injury stemming from any number of underlying causes including bacteria, yeast, and inflammation. This ointment needs to be ordered by a doctor or midwife and mixed by a pharmacist, usually in a compounding pharmacy. It is well absorbed into the skin and the baby will not take in very much at all. The mixture is to be used sparingly after each feeding and not wiped or washed off prior to nursings, although rinsing both nipples after nursing and before applying the ointment is still recommended by lactation consultants.

9. Bacteria in an open wound from the surrounding skin and hands can delay healing, and one study found that 75 percent of mothers with injured nipples at five days postpartum or beyond, usually from a faulty latch, develop mastitis in the coming weeks. Because so many mothers develop wounded nipples during the early days of nursing, I often recommend oral antibiotics to help the wound heal and prevent getting a breast infection later. If you have injured nipples at or after five days postpartum, call your midwife or obstetrician for a prescription of antibiotics.

Irritated nipples. Irritated nipples are reddened and sometimes slightly swollen, and generally they burn. Some mothers may feel burning between, as well as during, feedings. In severe cases, the nipples may be cracked, peeling, or oozing. Nipple irritation may be caused by yeast (thrush), bacteria, a chemical sensitivity or allergy, or a skin condition such as eczema or impetigo.

Thrush nipples. When a mother's nipples become sore after weeks or months of comfortable nursing, thrush (see page 108) is the usual cause. But a thrush infection can also occur in the early weeks after delivery, and when it does, it may be overlooked as the cause of the nipple soreness. A newborn with thrush may have picked up a yeast infection in the birth canal during delivery; this often happens if the mother is diabetic. A thrush infection may also result if a mother or her baby is given antibiotics (after a cesarean, antibiotics are often given in intravenous fluids).

If you suspect a case of thrush, carefully inspect the baby's mouth. You may see white patches on the inside of the cheeks, inside the lips, and possibly on the tongue. Sometimes a baby will have no symptoms in the mouth but will have a diaper rash caused by yeast. This rash, usually in the genital area, will be very defined, very red, and a bit raised. It may also appear in the folds of the baby's diaper area. There may be "satellite" areas apart from the main rash, and the rash may appear scaly. Another difference is that a yeast rash will not respond to typical remedies like frequent cleaning and the usual diaper rash creams. For treatment, see page 108.

Nipple Dermatitis. A slight reddening and a burning feeling in the nipples, in the absence of thrush or another underlying skin condition, usually indicate dermatitis. Nipple dermatitis can result from bacterial growth on the nipples or an allergy or sensitivity to a nipple cream or oil, laundry detergent, or fabric softener.

Common offenders are vitamin E preparations—oils, creams, or capsules. Mothers allergic to chocolate may develop an allergic reaction to preparations with cocoa butter, such as Balm Barr. Unmodified lanolin can also cause an allergic response, usually in a mother who is allergic to wool (from which lanolin comes) or very sensitive to it. Lanolin is found in pure hydrous and anhydrous forms and in many commercial creams, such as Massé breast cream, Mammol ointment, Eucerin, and A+D ointment. Modified lanolin, which has had the allergenic component removed, seldom causes allergic reactions.

Simply discontinuing use of the cream or oil, or switching to hypoallergenic detergents (free of perfumes and dyes), may bring relief, but usually additional measures are necessary.

TREATMENT MEASURES FOR NIPPLE DERMATITIS

1. You might try using Dr. Jack Newman's APNO on your nipples for a few days. See page 110.
2. Consult a doctor, preferably a dermatologist. Usually, a moderate- or high-strength anti-inflammatory cream and an antibiotic cream are prescribed.
3. Apply the medication to the irritated areas after every other nursing with clean hands, making sure your nipples are completely dry first. Apply the cream sparingly so that all of it is absorbed. If you see traces on your nipples when you are ready to nurse again, you are using too much. Dab the area with a tissue to absorb the excess.
4. Use the medication for as long as advised by your doctor. Although the pain may be gone in a day or two, the dermatitis may take from one to two weeks to completely heal.
5. Should you find that the medication aggravates your soreness, stop using it immediately. This may indicate that yeast is present and should be treated (see "Thrush Nipples," page 53).
6. Place cool, wet compresses on the nipples after nursing.
7. Review "General Comfort Measures for Sore Nipples," page 51.

Eczema and impetigo. Eczema can appear on the nipple and areola, making the area burn, itch, flake, ooze, or crust. Women with a history or current outbreak of eczema elsewhere on the body are most often affected. If you suspect eczema, seek treatment from a dermatologist.

Impetigo is a severe infection that causes continual sloughing off of the skin. When it occurs on the nipples, impetigo is very painful, but it can be quickly cured with an oral antibiotic or an antibiotic cream. Bactroban (mupirocin) is a prescription antibiotic cream commonly used to treat impetigo.

Breast Pain

Occasionally mothers complain of pain inside the breasts while nursing. You may feel pain in your breasts if you become engorged, which usually happens two to four days after delivery (see "Engorged Breasts," page 47). If your nipples are burning and pinker than normal, see "Irritated Nipples," page 53. If you feel a mild aching at the start of nursing, it may be related to the beginning of let-down.

Deep breast pains, sometimes described as "shooting," that occur soon after nursing may be related to the sudden refilling of the breast. These pains usually disappear after the first weeks of nursing. Shooting pain in the breast can also accompany plugged milk ducts (see page 112) and nipple irritation from yeast or dermatitis (see page 54).

Leaking Milk

During the early weeks of nursing, milk may drip, leak, or spray from the breasts. This is a normal sign of let-down. While the baby nurses at one breast, milk often drips or sprays from the other. Let-down, and leaking, may occur frequently and unexpectedly between nursings as well. Milk may leak during sleep. It may be stimulated by the baby's sounds, by thoughts about nursing, or by any routines associated with feeding time. A shower may stimulate let-down. Dripping, leaking, and spraying usually lessen considerably after a few weeks of nursing.

Some mothers' breasts do not leak. Women who have nursed previously may notice that their breasts leak less with subsequent children. Both of these situations are usually normal.

COPING MEASURES FOR LEAKING MILK

1. While nursing, open both bra flaps, and let the milk drip onto a small towel or diaper.
2. Change cloth or disposable nursing pads as soon as they become wet.
3. Try silicone LilyPadz, which don't absorb milk but instead apply a gentle pressure on the nipple to prevent leakage.
4. Avoid routine use of plastic breast shells if you do not need them to improve the shape of your nipples. They may keep your clothes dry, but they can cause excessive leaking and keep your nipples moist. Milk collected in the shells between nursings is unsafe for feeding. Only if the shells are washed just prior to nursing and put in place during nursing can the milk be stored for later feedings.
5. Don't try to control leaking by habitually pumping your breasts. Pumping actually stimulates greater milk production and could make your breasts fuller and more prone to leaking.
6. If your breasts leak during the night, place extra cloth or disposable pads in your bra or use silicone pads, which adhere to the skin and don't require a bra to hold them in place. Or simply spread a bath towel over the bed sheet to keep it and your mattress dry.

Let-Down Difficulty

During the early weeks of breastfeeding, the let-down response is developing. Sometimes mothers are told that they must be happy, relaxed, and carefree for the let-down of milk to occur. If this were the case, few women would ever succeed at nursing. Although many mothers worry that their milk won't be available as needed, let-down failure is extremely rare among women who nurse regularly and often.

For the establishment and maximal functioning of the let-down reflex, nurse the baby every two to three hours around the clock during the first week. Make sure that she is positioned correctly and is compressing the sinuses beneath the areola, and that her feeding time is not limited. Ideally, the baby should be allowed—encouraged, if necessary—to drain one or both breasts well at each feeding.

It is important to make yourself as comfortable as possible for feedings. The milk may not release completely if you are experiencing much pain—whether from sore nipples or from the trauma of delivery. Taking a mild pain reliever such as acetaminophen (Tylenol) or ibuprofen (Motrin, Advil) a half hour or so prior to nursing may help.

The signs of milk release during the first week will vary for each woman. They may include:

- Mild uterine cramping during nursing
- Increased vaginal flow during nursing
- Dripping, leaking, or spraying of milk, especially during nursing
- Occasional sensations in the breast during nursing
- Softening of the breasts after nursing

The most reliable indicator of milk let-down is the baby's swallowing. As the milk releases, the baby will swallow after every one or two sucks. Most women, particularly first-time mothers, do not feel the let-down reflex during the first few weeks after birth.

Usually when a mother believes she is experiencing a let-down difficulty, the problem is actually with the baby's latch-on or sucking or with a low milk supply. See "Difficult Latch-on: Refusal to Nurse," page 57; "Sucking Problems," page 69; and "Underfeeding and Weight Loss," page 73.

Milk Appearance

Whereas colostrum is usually clear, yellow, or orange, mature breast milk is white, sometimes with a bluish tint. If it resembles skim milk from the dairy, this does not mean your milk is "weak"; breast milk normally looks thin. Occasionally a mother discovers that her milk is green, blue, or pink. Such coloring is due to her intake of vegetables, fruits, food dyes, or dietary supplements and is not harmful to the baby.

Blood in the milk can usually be traced to a bleeding nipple. Occasionally, bleeding from the breast occurs during pregnancy or when breastfeeding begins. Frequently, a benign papilloma is the cause, and the bleeding generally stops within several days. Blood in the milk will not hurt the baby, though substantial amounts may make him vomit. If you are advised against nursing, pump for a few days. The problem will clear up on its own in a day or so.

Difficult Latch-On: Flat, Dimpled, or Inverted Nipples

Both mother and baby get frustrated when latching on to the breasts is difficult because of flat, dimpled, or inverted nipples. Typically, the problem is intensified if the breasts become engorged or overly full. When they do, even nipples that protruded before may suddenly flatten or dimple. Frequently, one nipple proves to be more troublesome than the other. Persistence and patience help most mothers through this problem.

Mothers with problem nipples are often more prone to soreness. This is because they tend to focus simply on getting the baby latched on rather than on getting the baby latched on well, with the nipple deep in the baby's mouth. A poor latch can lead to nipple soreness and even injury.

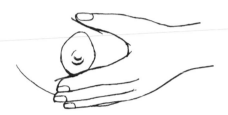

To help the baby latch on to an inverted nipple, place your thumb above the areola and your fingers below, and push your breast against your chest wall.

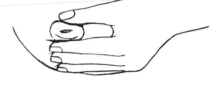

Don't squeeze your thumb and forefinger together, or the nipple may invert further.

TREATMENT MEASURES FOR FLAT, DIMPLED, OR INVERTED NIPPLES

1. Put the baby to the breast within the first two hours after birth. The timing of the first nursing may be critical when the nipples are flat, dimpled, or inverted. Many babies are able to latch on easily to problem nipples during this initial period, and they continue to do well.

2. To help the baby latch on to a flat nipple, make it stand out by pinching, stroking, or rolling it between your thumb and forefinger. Pinching a dimpled or inverted nipple could invert it further. To help the baby latch on to an inverted or dimpled nipple, place your thumb 1½ to 2 inches behind the nipple, with your fingers beneath, and pull back toward your chest. The crossover or football hold will allow you the most visibility and control. Consider trying "biological nurturing" (see page 34) to help the baby achieve a successful latch.

3. Express a few drops of colostrum or milk onto your nipple or onto the baby's lips if he is reluctant to latch on. Glucose water (available in hospital nurseries) dripped over the nipple may also entice the baby, although it sometimes makes the nipple

too slippery. At home, in a pinch, you can mix a teaspoon of refined sugar in a cup of warm boiled water, then drip the solution over your nipple. But never use regular honey or corn syrup on your nipple, as they have been associated with infant botulism.

4. Stop nursing if the baby is frantic. Expressing a few drops of colostrum or milk onto the baby's lips or dripping glucose water on his lips can help calm him and regain his interest in latching on.

5. If a nurse or another helper is working with you, try using the side-lying position—or, if you're large-breasted, the football hold—to allow your helper maximum visibility and control. If your nipples are dimpled or inverted, ask the helper to pull back on the breast behind the nipple rather than pinching it. Sometimes these sessions become intense and upsetting, so let your helper know when you or your baby needs a break. If you are in the hospital, let a variety of nurses or lactation professionals work with you; you can usually find one or two who are exceptionally skilled and sensitive.

Begin pumping and feeding by 24 hours after birth if your baby still has not latched on. A clinical-grade rental pump is usually the best choice for collecting milk and improving the nipple shape. Before the milk comes in, you may be able to collect even more colostrum by manually expressing it. You can read about manual expression and pumping on page 136. You can also learn the technique of hand expression from a lactation consultant or by viewing a helpful video made by Dr. Jane Morton of Stanford University at http://newborns.stanford.edu/Breastfeeding/HandExpression.html.

6. Continue putting the baby to breast.

7. Try to avoid giving the baby an artificial nipple of any kind for the first couple of days. Whether or not your baby has succeeded at latching on at first try, this may be very important. An artificial nipple can make his subsequent attempts at the breast more difficult. Options for feeding a newborn manually expressed or pumped colostrum include a dropper, a spoon, a syringe, and a soft cup.

8. Many mothers consider using a nipple shield when they have trouble getting their babies to latch on to the breast. A nipple shield is a thin, clear, soft silicone cover worn over the nipple. Holes at the tip allow milk to flow to the baby. When you use a shield, your baby may latch on and suck, but the sinuses behind the areola will not be adequately compressed unless the shield is the right size for both your nipple and the baby's mouth and the baby is well latched on to the breast and not just the shaft of the shield. Without expert help, a shield can thus inhibit the flow of milk and adequate emptying of the breast, which could lead to a poor milk supply and insufficient milk intake for the baby.

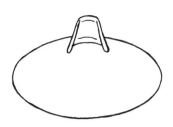

A nipple shield

If you want to try using a nipple shield to make your nipples stand out, wait until a couple of days after the birth, to give the baby a chance to learn to latch on without the shield and for your milk to come in. When using a shield, take it off after the baby has sucked for 1 to 2 minutes, and try to get him to latch on without it. Pumping just before nursing may work just as well as a nipple shield in making the nipples stand out. Use a nipple shield throughout feedings only if your milk is in and either (1) a lactation professional determines the correct shield size and makes sure that the baby is taking enough milk while you're wearing the shield, or (2) you use a clinical-grade rental pump after each nursing to guarantee that your breasts are being well emptied and also have the baby weighed every few days to make sure he is gaining at least an ounce a day.

9. If you and your baby are discharged from the hospital before nursing has occurred, locate a clinical-grade rental pump and use it at least eight times a day. (See chapter 5 for guidelines on pumping, and refer to the Appendix for the approximate amount of milk your baby needs at each feeding.) Keep trying to nurse; at least three or four short practice sessions per day, on a soft breast when the baby is not frantic, should eventually pay off.

10. If you become engorged when your milk comes in, soften the areola by pressing on it, as described on page 48. You can also try wearing breast shells in your bra for at least a half hour before nursing; this is often essential for dimpled or inverted nipples. Many hospital maternity units have breast shells. If yours doesn't, send your partner or a friend to a maternity shop or lactation clinic to purchase a pair. Lastly, you can briefly pump your breasts just before nursing to pull the nipples out enough for the baby to latch on.

If your baby continues to be unable to latch, there may come a time when it is best to begin feeding your milk by bottle. This may be when milk production begins and if it becomes too time-consuming to feed using other methods. In this situation, you may need a great deal of support and encouragement. Finding this support will make all the difference. Seeing a lactation professional may be very helpful. Remember that most insurance companies are required to cover lactation visits under the Affordable Care Act.

It is very common for a baby to suddenly latch on one day, rewarding his mother's persistence.

FATIGUE AND DEPRESSION

During this first week, make your life as simple as possible. Your partner or helper is essential to your recovery and adjustment. He or she can be most helpful in assuring your rest by taking over family and household duties and limiting phone calls and visitors.

Rest is necessary to your ability to cope during the postpartum period. Make a commitment to take at least one nap a day, to make up for sleep lost in labor and afterward. You may find that you are able to sleep better during naps and at night if you tuck the baby in with you. Babies often sleep better this way, too.

Turn off your cell phone, or mute it. An answering machine can be very helpful in preventing disruptions while you nap, if you adjust the number of rings. It's also handy when you are busy with nursing and baby care.

Eat a good breakfast; perhaps your partner can prepare it for you. If you lack an appetite at mealtimes, frequent snacking throughout the day on high-protein foods will assist your recovery and help maintain your energy level.

If you have had tearing or an episiotomy, or you have hemorrhoids, take several baths each day. Warm water is soothing and relaxing, and it will speed the healing of your perineum.

Don't expect to adjust to new parenthood on your own. Reach out for help or reassurance whenever you need it. Friends or relatives might welcome the opportunity to come and help out for a while, and you should feel free to call the hospital staff, a public health nurse, your childbirth instructor, or a breastfeeding counselor whenever you need assistance, reassurance, or support.

If you feel tired and overwhelmed, try not to keep it to yourself. Let your partner know; a good cry on someone's shoulder may leave you feeling much better. Avoid making your partner the target of your fears and anger. Instead of criticizing, let him know exactly what you need. One mother put it very well: "I just need him to give me hugs and let me know I'm doing okay." Your partner, after all, may be feeling as much stress as you are.

If you are alone with your baby during this first week, make a special effort to limit your activities. Perhaps you can have a friend come by to fix you lunch. Let the dishes soak all day, and tidy up the house for only 10 minutes at a time, if you must. Perhaps you can afford to pay for light housekeeping once or twice a week for a short period.

Feeling depressed over a birth experience is not uncommon. You may be able to resolve some of your feelings by talking to your childbirth instructor or birth attendant. In a week or two, you might try to locate a postpartum or cesarean support group.

CONCERNS ABOUT THE BABY

Sleepy Baby

Many babies are sleepy during the first several days after birth. They may be so sleepy that they refuse to wake for nursing or fall asleep after just a few minutes of sucking. Sleepiness during the first few days may be related in part to recovery following labor and delivery. Pain medications and general anesthetics given to the mother during the birth process also lessen the baby's wakefulness and interest in nursing. When newborns are wrapped snugly, too, they usually sleep for long periods of time (that's why nurses bundle them tightly). Babies may act too sleepy to nurse when they feel full from a water or formula supplement or an air bubble. The newborn with jaundice may also be somewhat sleepy.

Although it may seem unkind, after the first 24 hours the sleepy baby should be wakened and fed at least every two and a half hours (measured from the start of one nursing to the start of the next) during the day and evening, and every three to four hours in the night. The sleepy baby needs a "mother-led" rather than a "baby-led" schedule until she begins waking on her own. This is necessary not only for her nutritional well-being but also to ensure milk production and supply. Frequent feedings will also help minimize jaundice.

TREATMENT MEASURES FOR THE SLEEPY BABY

1. While in the hospital, take advantage of the baby's normal sleeping and waking cycles by keeping her with you as much as possible.
2. Avoid supplements, pacifiers, and nipple shields. All of these may decrease the baby's vigor at the breast.
3. Before attempting to nurse, wake the baby. Unwrap and undress her down to the diaper. Dim any bright lights, and sit the baby up on your lap by holding her under her chin. While talking to the baby, gently rub or pat her back (you may get a burp). Or place her against your bare chest and wait for her to begin rooting.
4. If the baby falls back asleep soon after latching on, massage or compress your breast to encourage more milk flow (see page 37). Babies are more vigorous at the breast when they are receiving milk.
5. Try the side-lying position; babies tend to nurse for longer periods in this position (get assistance, if needed, to help the baby latch on). The football hold can also be helpful in keeping a baby awake, though it is not as effective as side-lying.
6. Burp the baby after nursing at one breast to encourage her to take the other. Sitting the baby up in your lap and bending her slightly forward usually works best. If you don't get a burp after a couple of minutes, there is probably none to be had. Change her diaper if needed.
7. If all else fails, try again in an hour.
8. Alert your physician if your baby is very lethargic and cannot be roused by the preceding techniques after five to six hours.

Bowel Movements

Your baby's first few stools are called meconium. Meconium is black, greenish-black, or dark brown, and it's tarry or sticky. By the second or third day, after several good colostrum feedings, the baby will have passed most of the meconium. He may have a few greenish-brown or brownish-yellow transitional stools.

Once milk production is established and the baby is nursing well, stools take on their characteristic yellow or mustard color. This usually occurs by the fifth day, unless the baby is jaundiced and receiving phototherapy, which makes the stools dark, or is not getting enough milk. Yellow stools by the fifth day are usually a sign that the baby is getting sufficient milk.

During the early days most babies have at least two bowel movements daily. The stools of a breastfed baby are generally the consistency of yogurt. They are soft or even runny, and they may appear curdled or seedy. This is not diarrhea. These stools have a sweet or cheesy odor.

Your baby may pass his stools easily, or he may fuss, grunt, and turn red in the face while having a bowel movement. This is not constipation. Constipation is not possible as long as your baby is totally breastfed.

If your baby doesn't have bowel movements every day, or if by the fifth day his stools are still dark, he may not be getting enough milk. See "Underfeeding and Weight Loss," page 73, for more information on determining whether your baby is getting enough.

Jaundice

A yellowing of the skin and eyes, jaundice is caused by bilirubin, a yellow pigment that is present to some degree in all blood. The skin becomes yellowish when the amount of bilirubin is higher than normal. The

Bilirubin comes from the red blood cells. These cells live only a short time; as they are destroyed, bilirubin is made. Bilirubin is then processed through the liver and finally eliminated in the stool. During pregnancy, the mother's liver processes bilirubin for the baby. After birth, the baby's liver has to begin doing the job. This usually takes a few days. Until the baby's liver is able to process bilirubin, it may increase in the baby's blood. This normal rise is referred to as physiologic jaundice. This is the most common form of jaundice, and about 40 percent of all babies develop it. It is usually noticed on the second or third day of life, and it generally disappears by one week of age.

Mild to moderate jaundice of this type will not hurt a baby, although many parents worry about it. However, the baby who nurses poorly or not at all during the first few days may become jaundiced from the lack of colostrum, which is important for the elimination of meconium. When meconium is retained in the bowel longer than usual, bilirubin cannot be eliminated as needed. The best way to treat this jaundice is to make sure the baby gets plenty of colostrum and breast milk (see "Underfeeding and Weight Loss," page 73).

Some babies develop jaundice for other reasons. One type of jaundice, ABO incompatibility, occurs when the mother's blood type is O and the baby's blood type is A, B, or AB. During pregnancy, maternal antibodies cross the placenta, break down red blood cells, and cause more bilirubin to be produced in the baby after birth. On the first or second day after delivery, the bilirubin level may rise rapidly. Other, less common blood incompatibilities also produce elevated bilirubin levels. Babies of Asian descent typically experience higher bilirubin levels.

Babies with any bruises resulting from the birth process commonly develop jaundice. Also more prone to jaundice are babies who are sick right after birth or born prematurely, at low birth weights, or to diabetic mothers. Twins, too, are especially susceptible. Some drugs that are used during labor, including Pitocin, can also cause jaundice.

Another type of jaundice, common only to breastfed newborns, is known as breast-milk jaundice. It occurs in approximately one-third of all nursing babies, generally on the fifth day after birth. Breast-milk jaundice usually lasts four to six weeks but can continue for as long as eight to ten weeks. When a baby's skin stays yellow beyond the first week, breast-milk jaundice is diagnosed by laboratory tests to rule out other forms of jaundice. Breastfeeding need not be interrupted to make this diagnosis. The exact cause of this jaundice is still unknown, but it has never been known to cause any problem for a baby.

If your baby looks jaundiced, the doctor may order tests to measure the level of bilirubin in the blood and determine whether treatment is necessary. If the baby was born at term and is otherwise healthy, many doctors will not order treatment unless the bilirubin level is over 20 milligrams per deciliter. Frequent breastfeeding may be all that is necessary.

Some jaundiced babies are treated with phototherapy. The "bili-lights," along with frequent nursing, help to destroy excess bilirubin. The baby usually lies under these lights from two to four days, her eyes covered with a protective mask.

Often the bilirubin level will stay constant for 24 hours but drop by 48 hours. The treatment is discontinued as soon as the bilirubin level has dropped to a normal level. Usually a baby is hospitalized for phototherapy, but in some communities home phototherapy services are available.

Rarely, usually in cases of blood incompatibility, the bilirubin climbs rapidly to high levels. On these occasions an exchange transfusion may be done to reduce the bilirubin. Over an hour or two, small amounts of the baby's blood are taken out and replaced with donated blood.

Some doctors ask the mother to stop breastfeeding temporarily whenever a baby becomes jaundiced. This is generally unwise, since breastfeeding is usually one of the most effective ways of eliminating jaundice. Calling a halt to nursing is also unfortunate for the mother, who may wonder if her milk is really best for her baby.

Mothers are also commonly told that their nursing babies need water supplements to help get rid of jaundice. But water supplements do not lower the level of bilirubin in the blood. Some studies suggest, in fact, that water supplements are associated with higher bilirubin levels. In addition, babies who are routinely given water tend to be nursed less frequently, and they have a higher rate of early weaning.

Since 1994, the American Academy of Pediatrics has recommended a different approach: Healthy, full-term babies over 72 hours old with bilirubin levels below 20 milligrams per deciliter (or 340 micromoles per liter) should be nursed frequently, at least eight times every 24 hours, and should receive no water supplements.

1. Let the baby's physician know you prefer to continue nursing throughout the period of jaundice.

2. Nurse frequently, ideally every two to two and a half hours, and encourage the baby to suck for at least 15 to 20 minutes at each breast. If your baby needs phototherapy, taking her from under the bili-light for these feedings will not delay the effectiveness of treatment. Intermittent phototherapy is thought to be as effective as continuous exposure.

3. If your baby is sleepy, as jaundiced babies sometimes are, see "Sleepy Baby," page 61, for effective measures to wake her for feedings.

4. Avoid water supplements, as these do not reduce bilirubin levels and may discourage the baby from nursing frequently.

5. To be sure your baby is getting enough milk, keep track of her bowel movements. She should have at least two each day, and preferably three or more. She should have lost less than 10 percent of her birth weight, and she should gain an ounce a day after the fifth day. If she isn't gaining this much, refer to "Underfeeding and Weight Loss," page 73.

6. If you are still hospitalized or you are welcome to stay in a hospital room while your baby is being treated, ask the nurses if you can have the baby's crib and light set up next to your bed so you can care for the baby and nurse frequently.

7. If you cannot stay 24 hours a day with your baby, express your milk every three hours using a clinical-grade rental pump (see page 140 for advice on pumping). Take your milk to the hospital for the feedings you will miss.

8. If your doctor is firm in his or her desire for you to temporarily stop nursing, again, express your milk every three hours to keep up your supply. Freeze your milk, and save it for later.

9. If you are struggling to get your baby to latch on, you may find that she becomes upset even when you bring her near your breast. In this situation, you may begin to think that your baby does not want to nurse. Nothing could be further from the truth. If your baby cries at the breast and seems unwilling to try to latch on, know that she is simply frustrated. She is crying because she wants to latch on and suck but isn't getting the signal she needs. She cannot feel your nipple far enough back in her mouth.

Difficult Latch-On: Refusal to Nurse

Latch-on problems can originate either with the baby or with the mother. Some babies fail to latch on well because they are sleepy (see "Sleepy Baby," page 61). Many babies struggle to latch on when the breast becomes overly full or engorged (see "Engorged Breasts," page 47), when the mother and baby are not positioned well for latch-on, or when the mother has flat, dimpled, or inverted nipples (see "Difficult Latch-on: Flat, Dimpled, or Inverted Nipples," page 57). Problems other than these are as follows.

The baby who has nursed earlier. During the first week, a baby who has already nursed may suddenly refuse one or both sides. He may simply act uninterested although he is awake, or he may become upset when put to one or both breasts. This may be because he has been given a bottle or pacifier during the first week and has developed a preference for an artificial nipple. Such a baby will likely start nursing again after a few hours un-coaxed or after one or more of the following measures are taken.

TREATMENT MEASURES FOR THE BABY WHO STOPS NURSING

1. If you are overly full or engorged, soften the areola by pressing it (see page 37) or by manually expressing or pumping a little milk (see chapter 5) just before putting the baby to breast.
2. If the baby is frantic, calm him. A few drops of colostrum or glucose water dripped on his lips or over the nipple may alert and encourage him. Glucose water is available only in hospital nurseries, but at home, in a pinch, you can mix a teaspoon of refined sugar in a cup of warm boiled water to entice the baby. Occasionally a very upset baby may need to be tightly swaddled in a thin blanket.
3. Pay attention to proper positioning (see "Positioning at the Breast," page 29). When the baby turns his face from side to side with his mouth wide open, pull him in closer so his tongue can feel the nipple. Consider trying "biological nurturing" (see page 34) to see if the baby can achieve a successful latch more easily in this position.
4. Try letting the baby suck on your finger for a few seconds just before putting him to breast.
5. If the baby seems to spit out the nipple with his tongue, try holding some covered ice against the nipple for a few minutes to firm it. This can be particularly effective for the baby who has become used to an artificial nipple.
6. Persist. The baby who is hiccuping, having a bowel movement, or staring at his mother or something else interesting will usually be reluctant to latch on. Try again in an hour or so.
7. Coax the baby who is suddenly refusing one breast by using the football hold on that side.
8. If you can't get the baby latched on, express your milk until you can, using a clinical-grade rental pump. This may be crucial to bringing in your milk supply and to maintaining high production. Refer to chapter 5, for information on pumping milk, and the Appendix for the approximate amounts of milk a baby needs at each feeding.
9. Get a lot of support and encouragement. If possible, see a lactation professional.

The baby who refuses one side. Some babies latch easily to one side but refuse the other. This may happen when one nipple is more difficult for her because of the nipple size or shape (see "Difficult Latch-on: Flat, Dimpled, or Inverted Nipples," page 57). Some babies may feel uncomfortable lying on one side. This can happen when a baby has a fairly common condition known as torticollis. Torticollis can be present at birth or take up to three months to develop, and most doctors believe it could be related to abnormal positioning of the fetus inside the uterus. This condition puts pressure on a baby's sternocleidomas-toid muscle, the large muscle that runs on both sides of the neck from the back of the ears to the collarbone. Extra pressure on one side of this muscle can cause it to tighten, making it difficult for a baby to turn his neck. Babies with torticollis will act like most other babies except when it comes to activities that involve turning. A baby with torticollis keeps his head in one direction when lying down and tilts the head in just one direction, and has difficulty nursing on one side. If you think your baby might have torticollis, ask your doctor to examine your baby, which involves seeing how far your baby can turn his head. If a diagnosis is made, the doctor will probably teach you neck stretching exercises to practice with your baby at home. These exercises help loosen the tight muscle and strengthen the weaker one on the opposite side. This will help straighten out your baby's neck. In certain cases, the doctor may suggest taking your baby to a physical therapist for more intensive treatment. In the meantime, you may need to position your baby differently—for instance, using the football hold—for him to be able to latch on to the breast.

The baby who has not yet nursed. If a day or more has passed since the baby's birth and she still has not managed to latch on and suck, she may have one of the specific problems described as follows.

Recessed jaw. Some babies are born with a very recessed lower jaw. This can best be seen by looking at the baby's face in profile. A recessed jaw is problematic because a baby can latch on only if her chin reaches the breast before her upper lip; otherwise she can't take enough breast tissue into her mouth.

When you try to get a baby like this to latch on, make sure your breast isn't overly full. Extend the baby's head slightly backward as you bring her onto the breast so that her chin touches the breast first. Consider trying "biological nurturing" (see page 34) to see if the baby can latch on to the breast in this position. A baby with a recessed jaw will probably begin latching on and sucking between four and six weeks of age. In the meantime, you may need to pump your milk and feed it to your baby by bottle.

Tongue-tied. Some infants who can't latch on to the breast—mostly males—are tongue-tied. This means that the frenulum, or string-like tissue that attaches to the underside of the tongue, is so short or connected so close to the tip of the tongue that the baby may not be able to extend his tongue past his bottom lip. More important, he may not be able to raise his tongue high enough to express the milk from the breast. Although he may be able to suck on a finger or rubber nipple that extends well into his mouth, he may be unable to grasp the underside of his mother's nipple. Not only does he fail to get milk, but nursing may be very painful for his mother even when the baby is correctly positioned. Sometimes a clicking sound can be heard as the baby sucks. Occasionally a tongue-tied baby can manage to latch on to one breast but not the other.

The solution is simple: the frenulum should be clipped to release the tongue. Some physicians are reluctant or unwilling to perform this procedure, called a frenotomy, because studies conducted many years ago showed that tongue-tied infants rarely de-

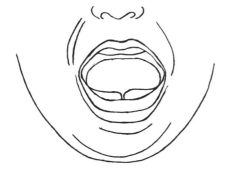

The tongue-tied baby may not be able to extend his tongue far enough or high enough to latch on to his mother's nipple.

veloped speech difficulties later in life; the studies concluded that tongue clipping was therefore unnecessary. Unfortunately, though, some tongue-tied babies are unable to breastfeed. If you cannot persuade your doctor to clip the frenulum, find another who will. A surgeon or dentist may do this in his office, and the procedure takes just a minute. You can see Dr. Jane Morton's photographs of a baby both before and after a frenotomy by following the link at http://newborns.stanford.edu/Frenotomy.html. Dr. Bobby Ghaheri's website also contains a wealth of information and resources for nursing the tongue-tied baby: www.drghaheri.squarespace.com.

Upper lip tie. Some newborns are born with their upper lip "tied" to their upper gum. Usually this poses no problems with nursings. If severe, it can cause the baby's upper lip to turn inward instead of outward. This may be irritating to the nipple if severe enough. Few pediatricians recognize this problem, but some pediatric dentists believe that an upper lip tie can lead to a gap between the teeth later on or can cause a problem with dental decay. If it seems to be causing nursing pain, an evaluation with a pediatric dentist may be in order. Again, Dr. Ghaheri's website may be helpful.

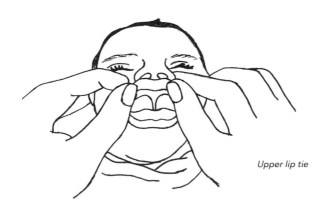

Upper lip tie

Protruding tongue. A few babies have tongues that protrude. The tongue may look longer than normal; it may be visible between the lips much of the time. Some mothers have described the protruding tongue as forming a hump in the mouth that the nipple is not able to get past.

You may be able to teach the baby to nurse by encouraging her to open wide with her tongue down and pulling back behind the areola just before latch-on. The football hold is recommended for the best visibility and control.

If you manage to get the baby onto the breast, be sure she is sucking adequately. This means she does not come off the breast easily; she is taking long, drawing sucks; and she is audibly swallowing.

Tongue sucking. Other infants who have difficulty latching on to the breast are those who suck their own tongues. These babies usually slide off the nipple after one or two sucks, and their cheeks dimple with each suck. They may also make clicking noises. When the baby opens her mouth to root or to cry, you may notice that her tongue is far back in her mouth or is curled toward the roof of her mouth.

Attempt to get the baby to latch on only when she opens wide with her tongue down. Stimulating the lower lip or slightly depressing the chin may help the tongue to drop. Pull the baby in close. The crossover or football hold is best when you are alone, and side-lying will give more control and visibility when someone is assisting you.

When refusal persists. If you have followed the preceding suggestions and your baby still has not latched on, try the following measures.

TREATMENT MEASURES FOR REFUSAL TO NURSE

1. Work with the baby in short, frequent sessions. If someone is assisting you, the side-lying position may give the greatest control and visibility. These sessions may become intense and upsetting for both you and the baby, so let your helper know if you need a break. If you are in the hospital, ask for help from various nurses or lactation professionals. You may find one or two who are exceptionally skilled and sensitive.

2. Encourage your baby by expressing a few drops of milk onto your nipple or onto his lips. Or try glucose water (available in the hospital) or, at home, a teaspoon of sugar—never corn syrup or honey—in a cup of warm boiled water (see page 57).

3. Try "biological nurturing" (see page 34) to see if the baby will latch on in this position.

4. If, 24 hours after birth, your baby still has not latched on, begin manually expressing or pumping (see page 136) and feeding the baby your expressed colostrum. But don't feed it by bottle; an artificial nipple of any kind could make his attempts at the breast more difficult. Alternatives to a bottle are a dropper, a spoon, a syringe, and a soft cup. Express your colostrum and feed it to the baby at least eight times in each 24 hours.

5. Continue pumping and feeding at least eight times in each 24 hours.

6. If your baby "shuts down" or gets upset at the breast, let him suck on a finger, nail side down. After a minute or two, quickly offer the breast, compressing it tightly so that it extends as far as possible into the baby's mouth.

7. Pump just before nursing to make your nipples stand out more. Some babies do better on a soft or half-empty breast.

8. If you use a nipple shield to help the baby latch on (see page 58), take it off after the baby has sucked for 1 to 2 minutes, and try to get him to latch on without it. Use a nipple shield throughout feedings only if your milk is in and either (1) a lactation professional has determined the correct shield size and made sure that the baby is taking enough milk while you're wearing the shield, or (2) you use a clinical-grade rental pump after each nursing to guarantee that your breasts are being well emptied, and you have the baby weighed every few days to make sure he is gaining at least an ounce a day.

9. If your baby seems to latch on but sucks only once or twice, he is probably not well attached. Take him off the breast and try again.

10. Continue short practice nursing sessions several times a day. Try to be patient but persistent; don't give up on your baby.

11. If your baby continues to refuse to nurse, there may come a time when it is best to begin feeding your pumped milk by bottle. This may be when milk production begins, if it becomes too time-consuming to feed using other methods.

12. Get a lot of support and encouragement. Ideally, see a lactation professional. Your insurance should cover this.

Many babies with latch-on problems overcome them during the first ten days, but a significant number first latch on at about one month of age. With this in mind, know that the most important thing to do until the baby finally latches is to keep your milk production as high as possible. See chapter 5 for advice on how to do this.

Sucking Problems

Some babies seem to latch on to the breast well but suck poorly. With some, the suction is so poor that they easily slide off the breast or can be taken off effortlessly. A baby's cheeks may dimple with each suck, and frequent clicking noises may be audible. Such a baby isn't really sucking on the nipple but on her tongue, which may perhaps be a habit developed in the uterus. Other babies with poor suction may have one of the physical problems described under "The Baby Who Has Not Yet Nursed," page 66. Babies with poor suction receive only the milk that drips into their mouths.

Although most babies with sucking problems have them from birth, others may develop them if they lose much weight, usually close to a pound, by the end of the first week. If this happens, and the baby cannot correct her suck after several good attempts at latching on, express your milk and feed it to her for 24 to 72 hours, supplementing breast milk with formula as necessary. After the baby is rehydrated and has regained a few ounces, she may correct her suck on her own.

A baby may have difficulty sucking at one or both breasts because he is tongue-tied. In this situation, the tongue is tethered by the short piece of tissue beneath. No matter how hard the baby tries, he isn't able to reach his tongue forward and then up far enough to strip the milk from the breast. Not only may he fail to get milk, but nursing a tongue-tied baby may be very painful for the mother, even when the baby is correctly positioned. Sometimes a clicking sound can be heard as the baby sucks. To correct the problem, have your baby's doctor or dentist clip the baby's frenulum (see page 66).

Another group of babies who have difficulty sucking and getting enough milk are those with very high palates. When the roof of the mouth is very high, the baby has trouble compressing the breast against the palate to express the milk into her mouth. Many babies with high, arched palates do little swallowing at the breast and fail to gain weight well. Few health professionals, including pediatricians, yet recognize high palates as a potential problem for nursing babies. If it is difficult to see the very top of a baby's palate without placing your head close to the baby's chest, or if the shape of the roof looks much deeper than the curve of a teaspoon, the palate may be too high. If you can get the baby to suck on your little finger (nail side down), and you feel a frequent loss of suction between your finger and his tongue, or your finger isn't in firm contact with the roof of his mouth, the palate may be too high. Another sign of a high palate may be clicking sounds while the baby is sucking.

In the case of a high palate, the mother should use an electric pump right after each nursing to bolster her milk supply. After a few days the baby will usually start to swallow more at the breast and gain weight better, but as soon as the pumping stops, the baby may begin to take less milk and will again fail to gain sufficient weight. Usually supple-mental pumping is necessary for several weeks, until the baby has grown enough to suck more efficiently. Using the football hold, or positioning the baby straddling your thigh, may help the baby suck better. Time is often the remedy for babies with sucking problems.

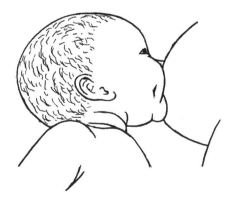

Dimpling of the baby's cheeks during nursing may signify an inadequate suck.

Lastly, babies whose mothers have large nipples—as large as or larger than a quarter—may be unable to suck effectively. Instead of latching on to the areola, behind the nipple, the baby compresses only the nipple itself, and so gets very little milk. In this case the mother needs to express her milk, using a clinical-grade rental pump, to build and maintain high production until the baby has grown enough to latch on to and compress the breast, not just the nipple. The mother will also need to obtain a large flange for effective pumping (see page 145).

TREATMENT MEASURES FOR THE BABY WITH POOR SUCKING

1. Remove the baby from the breast as soon as the faulty suck is evident.
2. Check the position of the tongue when the baby's mouth is wide open. If the tongue is curled against the roof of the mouth, try to lower it with your finger by stimulating the lower lip.
3. Using the crossover or football hold, compress the breast behind the nipple, and pull the baby in as close as possible for latch-on.
4. Try "biological nurturing" (see page 34) to see if the baby can achieve better suction in this position.
5. Work with the baby in short, frequent sessions. If someone is assisting you, the side-lying position may give the greatest control and visibility. These sessions may become intense and upsetting for both you and the baby, so let your helper know if you need a break.
6. If, 24 hours after birth, your baby still is not sucking well, begin manually expressing or pumping (see page 136) and feeding the baby your expressed colostrum. But don't feed it by bottle; an artificial nipple of any kind could make his attempts at the breast more difficult. Alternatives to a bottle are a dropper, a spoon, a syringe, and a soft cup. Express your colostrum and feed it to the baby at least eight times in each 24 hours.
7. Try manually expressing or pumping just before nursing. Some babies do better on a soft or half-empty breast.
8. If you use a nipple shield to help the baby latch on (see page 58), take it off after the baby has sucked for 1 to 2 minutes, and try to get him to latch on without it. Use a nipple shield throughout feedings only if your milk is in and either (1) a lactation professional has determined the correct shield size and made sure that the baby is taking enough milk while you're wearing the shield, or (2) you use a clinical-grade rental pump after each nursing to guarantee that your breasts are being well emptied, and you have the baby weighed every few days to make sure he is gaining at least an ounce a day.
9. Continue short practice nursing sessions several times a day. Try to be patient but persistent; don't give up on your baby.
10. If your baby continues to have sucking problems, there may come a time when it is best to begin feeding your pumped milk by bottle. This may be when milk production begins, if it becomes too time-consuming to feed using other methods.

11. If you are discharged from the hospital and the baby still isn't nursing well, use a clinical-grade rental pump (see page 140) for collecting your milk. Continue pumping your milk and feeding it to the baby at least eight times in each 24 hours.

12. Get a lot of support and encouragement. Make an appointment to see a lactation professional. Your insurance carrier should cover visits with a lactation consultant for you and your baby.

Like babies with latch-on problems, those with sucking problems often overcome them during the first ten days, but many improve only at about four to six weeks of age. With this in mind, know that the most important thing to do until the baby finally overcomes the problem is to keep your milk production as high as possible. See chapter 5 for advice on how to do this.

Fussiness and Excessive Night Waking

It can come as a surprise when your baby suddenly becomes fussy after spending most of his first few days sleeping. It is difficult to listen to your baby's cry; it may feel like an alarm going off in your body. Sometimes parents are told it is healthy for babies to cry or that babies will become spoiled if tended to every time they fuss. But comforting your infant and responding to her needs is very important to her well-being and her development of trust. Babies are really unspoilable.

Newborns cry for a variety of reasons. Often they are fussy during the first night home from the hospital. They may be hungry as often as every hour, especially when your milk is just starting to come in, or when feedings have been limited because of their sleepiness or for other reasons. Some babies seem to need more sucking time than others. Some seem to pass a lot of gas, which causes them discomfort. Many newborns become upset when they are not kept snugly wrapped. Perhaps they miss the close, secure feeling of the womb.

Then there are the babies who sleep most of the day and wake frequently during the night. These babies are said to have their days and nights mixed up.

COPING MEASURES FOR FUSSINESS

1. Nurse your baby on demand, approximately every two to three hours for at least 10 to 20 minutes at each breast.

2. Massage or compress your breasts while you nurse to increase the flow of milk (see page 37).

3. Burp the baby after he finishes at each breast.

4. Wrap the baby snugly in a light blanket after each feeding.

5. Avoid water or formula supplements.

6. If the baby seems unsatisfied after a feeding, nurse him some more, or rock him or walk with him next to your body and then nurse him again in an hour or two.

7. If the baby frequently seems discontent after nursings, refer to "Underfeeding and Weight Loss," page 73.

Newborns normally wake about every three hours during the night. If your baby wakes more often than this, nurse her more often during the daytime and evening, every two to two and a half hours. If the baby has been sleeping through feeding times, wake her. See "Sleepy Baby," page 61.

Your baby may be crying at night not because she is hungry but because she wants to be close to you. Try tucking her in with you for at least a few nights. You may both sleep better.

Underfeeding and Weight Loss

During the first week, you may wonder if your baby is getting enough to eat. You may worry about whether your milk is adequate—especially if the baby seems to be nursing all the time or is fussy after feedings. Some mothers wonder if their milk has dried up when they observe the normal softening of the breast that occurs as the initial engorgement recedes.

Seeing if the baby will take a bottle of water or formula after nursing is not a reliable method of determining whether he is getting enough breast milk. Most babies will take a couple of ounces of water or formula if it is offered, even when they have had enough milk from the breast.

A baby can lose too much weight, though, when the milk doesn't come in by the third or fourth day, when nursing is infrequent, or when he has had trouble latching on and nursing well during the period of initial engorgement. Excessive weight loss can also occur when a mother uses a nipple shield over her nipple for nursing, when a newborn has a faulty suck, and, certainly, when a baby is sick. Babies who have high palates or who are tongue-tied may fail to express milk well while nursing and thus get too little milk (see "Sucking Problems," page 69). Other women who may be unable to produce enough milk are those with insufficient glandular (milk-producing) tissue, or hypoplastic breasts (see page 146), and some with polycystic ovary syndrome, or PCOS. Sometimes laxatives the mother has taken can cause a baby to have excessive bowel movements and to lose weight or gain too slowly.

Signs of adequate milk intake are listed on page 39. If you and your baby don't show all these signs, have him weighed. If you find that your baby has lost 10 percent or more of his birth weight within the first five days after birth, or if he isn't gaining an ounce per day after the fifth day, take the following measures.

TREATMENT MEASURES FOR UNDERFEEDING

1. See a lactation professional. Again, your insurance provider should cover these services.
2. To estimate the amount of milk you are producing and to increase your milk supply, obtain a clinical-grade rental breast pump (see chapter 5). Any other pump might be inadequate for estimating milk production and rebuilding a low milk supply. To estimate your milk production, pump immediately after nursing the baby. If you have a double collection kit, which is ideal, pump for a total of 10 to 20 minutes, or

longer if the milk continues to flow. If you are pumping one breast at a time, pump each twice, for a total pumping time of 20 to 30 minutes, or longer if the milk is still flowing. Feed your baby this milk and any necessary formula.

Exactly two hours after completing this pumping, pump again instead of nursing. You may very well get less milk at this second pumping than at the first. Multiply the number of ounces collected at the second pumping by 12. This will give you an estimate of how much milk you are producing over a 24-hour period; if you collect 1½ ounces, for example, you are producing about 18 ounces per day.

3. Offer the pumped milk to the baby. If you determine that you have enough milk for your baby and yet she has not been gaining well, it may be that she is not taking all of the milk available at some or many of her feedings. This can happen with newborns who were born prematurely, who tend to drift off to sleep while nursing, or who have sucking difficulties.

4. Review the video recommended in chapter 2 to be sure your baby is latching on well. Consider using "biological nurturing" (see page 34) to see if she can achieve a deeper latch this way.

5. Nurse at least eight times in every 24 hours, even if this means waking the baby for feedings (see "Sleepy Baby," page 61). Nurse for 10 to 15 minutes at each breast, or for as long as the baby is swallowing. If the baby swallows for only a few minutes, compress your breast (see page 37) to increase the flow. You can also switch the baby from breast to breast each time the swallowing stops.

6. If you're not producing as much milk as your baby needs, stimulate greater milk production by pumping your breasts right after each nursing. Pumping both breasts at the same time not only takes less time but is more effective in stimulating increased milk production. Use a double collection kit, if you have one, for 5 to 10 minutes, or pump each breast separately for 5 minutes, and then return to each breast a second time for a few more minutes. You can also spend a few minutes hand-expressing milk from both breasts after pumping to help insure more complete emptying (see page 136). After pumping, feed the baby whatever breast milk you've collected, along with formula as necessary.

7. If the baby needs supplemental formula, divide the amount of supplement needed daily by the number of feedings the baby is getting each day (usually eight). A baby who needs 3½ ounces of formula, for example, should get a bit less than ½ ounce after each of her eight daily nursings. The goal is to offer about the same amount of breast milk and formula at each feeding so that the baby wants to nurse at regular intervals.

8. Some mothers consider using donated breast milk from friends, relatives, or even strangers. For more information on the possible risks of using donated milk, see page 50.

9. Consider using herbs to stimulate greater milk production (see page 50).

10. Ignore any suggestions to drink a beer or two to help increase milk production. Drinking beer can in fact lessen milk production.

11. If your milk production remains low even with the use of herbs, talk to your doctor about using a pharmaceutical drug, like domperidone, to stimulate more production.

12. As long as you must provide supplemental feedings, find a method that suits you. Many lactation professionals, fearing that bottle-feeding might interfere with the baby's ability at the breast, suggest using a nursing supplementer, a cup, a soft tube with a syringe or finger, or an eyedropper. If one of these methods is recommended to you and it works well, good. But if you find it too frustrating or time-consuming, use a bottle. After the first few days of breastfeeding, supplementing by bottle rarely causes "nipple confusion."

13. Weigh your baby every few days to make sure that she is gaining well.

14. After each weighing, re-estimate your baby's milk needs. Then, two hours after your most recent pumping, express your milk instead of nursing and re-estimate your milk production (see step 2). If your production has increased enough to match the baby's needs, you can decrease or even eliminate any formula supplementation.

15. Consider renting a highly accurate electronic baby scale. Use the scale before and after feedings to determine how much milk the baby takes from the breast. One gram of weight increase is equal to one milliliter of milk intake.

16. Once your baby is gaining well, her nursing seems more vigorous, and you are supplementing nursings only with your breast milk, you might try eliminating some of the supplement. For a few days, offer the baby only half of the milk that you are expressing, and freeze the rest. If the baby gains well over these few days, continue pumping, but don't offer her any of the expressed milk. If the baby continues to gain an ounce a day without any supplement, gradually stop pumping. Continue to have your baby weighed weekly.

If treatment fails. Although the technique just outlined will normally reverse a case of underfeeding within a few days, sometimes, when breast engorgement has been severe and little milk has been removed during this critical period, the decline in milk production can be difficult to reverse. In unusual instances, a mother fails to produce enough milk even after weeks of both stepped-up nursing and pumping. This can occur if the placenta was not completely delivered at the time of the birth (see page 48). It sometimes happens to women who have had breast surgery, particularly if the surgical incision was made around the areola. Other women who may be unable to produce enough milk are those with insufficient glandular (milk-producing) tissue, or hypoplastic breasts, and some with polycystic ovary syndrome, or PCOS.

In any of these situations, lack of support from family, friends, and health professionals can make matters worse. But even with all of the best information and support, things sometimes don't turn out as we hope. If after giving breastfeeding your best effort you end up having to feed formula, you have not failed as a mother. Be proud of your efforts to nurse, and concentrate on providing your baby with all of the cuddling and loving that you can. Detailed information about formula and bottle-feeding can be found in *The Nursing Mother's Guide to Weaning* (see "Suggested Supplemental Reading," page 182).

Some mothers with insufficient milk production have found that continuing to nurse with a nursing supplementer has been a rewarding experience. Others have found nursing supplementers to be cumbersome and frustrating. Another option, particularly if the baby has become frustrated at the breast, is to bottle-feed and then nurse. "Comfort nursing"—nursing just after bottle-feedings, in between bottle-feedings, or during the night—may be a pleasant experience for both mother and baby.

DRUGS THAT STIMULATE MILK PRODUCTION

Two pharmaceutical drugs used to help build the milk supply are metoclopramide (Reglan) and domperidone.

Metoclopramide is prescribed in the United States primarily for gastric reflux. But several studies have shown it to be effective and safe for increasing a mother's milk supply, although the U.S. Food and Drug Administration (FDA) has not approved the drug for this use. Metoclopramide has not been shown to cause any problems for a nursing baby; in fact, it is occasionally prescribed for infants. It may, however, make the mother sleepy. More worrisome side effects, such as agitation and uncontrolled muscle movements, are uncommon; if they occur, the drug should be discontinued. The typical dosage is 10 milligrams every six to eight hours for 14 days. If taken for longer than a few weeks, metoclopramide can lead to depression and other problems that may not resolve simply by discontinuing the medication. It should therefore never be taken for more than two to four weeks.

Although domperidone is marketed only for gastrointestinal disorders, studies show that it safely increases milk production, and the American Academy of Pediatrics has approved this drug, as well as metoclopramide, as safe to take while nursing. Domperidone apparently works by stimulating production of prolactin, the hormone that stimulates the breast to produce milk.

Because domperidone does not enter the brain tissue in significant amounts, it has far less frequent and serious side effects in the nursing mother than does metoclopramide. The side effects that can occur—headache, abdominal cramps, and dry mouth—are extremely uncommon when the drug is taken orally in normal doses for stimulating milk production, no higher than 40 milligrams four times per day. (The FDA issued a warning about domperidone after reports of sickness when the drug was administered in high intravenous doses as treatment for gastrointestinal disturbances. According to Thomas Hale, a professor of pediatrics and pharmacology at Texas Tech University School of Medicine, this use of the drug caused blood levels 80 to 150 times higher than that of women who take domperidone orally in normal doses.)

Although domperidone is not manufactured in the United States, it can be made here in compounding pharmacies, which operate in most areas. But the drug is much less expensive, and available without a prescription, when ordered through InHouse Pharmacy in Vanuatu.

Special Babies

NURSING CAN BE A SPECIAL CHALLENGE in certain circumstances—situations that may result from a long-standing condition or that may take you completely by surprise. Either way, you may be tempted to give up the idea of breastfeeding altogether. The specific guidelines in this chapter should help you make a realistic appraisal of your situation and find, I hope, the happiest solution for you and your baby.

NURSING AN ADOPTED BABY

More and more mothers who are planning to adopt babies are considering breastfeeding them. An infant's suck can stimulate milk production whether or not the mother has ever had or nursed a baby before, and even if she has reached menopause. Most adoptive mothers, however, need to supplement their breast milk, many for the entire time they are nursing. Probably the safest and most convenient way to supplement breastfeeding is with a nursing supplementation device specifically designed for this situation.

Some women's enthusiastic claims of producing abundant milk for their adopted babies may set up other adoptive mothers for disappointment. It is impossible to predict whether an adoptive mother will be able to produce milk, or how much she will produce, even if she is currently nursing or has recently nursed another baby. Adoptive nursing will be most successful if you focus on the relationship between you and your baby, rather than on your milk production. Measure your success by whether the experience truly helps make the baby yours.

Before the baby arrives, it is wise to learn as much as possible about breastfeeding and adoptive nursing. Be sure that the pediatrician you're choosing for your baby will be supportive of your efforts. A lactation professional may be able to refer you to other adoptive mothers who have nursed their babies.

Nursing an adopted baby doesn't require any advance preparation; you can simply put the baby to the breast and see what happens. In this case, though, you may or may not eventually produce significant amounts of breast milk. But if you know at least several weeks in advance that your baby is coming, you may be able to increase your chance of producing ample milk by following one of the treatment plans developed by Jack Newman, a physician, and Lenore Goldfarb, a lactation professional. When your baby arrives, he may be easily persuaded to begin nursing, or he may require a great deal of patience and persistence. In general, the younger the baby is, the easier the transition from the bottle to the breast will be. See page 00 for assistance in getting the baby to nurse.

Most adoptive mothers need to supplement their milk with formula. Some women try to increase their milk production by using formula in only minimal amounts or by overdiluting it. But these practices often result in stress and underfeeding for the baby.

If you've decided to use a supplementation device, you may be hoping for donations of breast milk to use in it, and perhaps you've already received offers of donated milk. But don't expect others to continue donating indefinitely. It can be a real effort for a nursing mother to collect extra milk. There is also the remote possibility that infectious diseases, including HIV and hepatitis, could be transmitted through donated milk.

Women who have breastfed adopted children often say that it has been one of the most memorable and rewarding experiences of their lives. You may especially enjoy nursing your adopted baby when she is older and you needn't concern yourself so much about milk production. Moments spent soothing a tired, hurt, or frustrated baby or toddler at the breast are priceless for any nursing mother.

MEDICAL REASONS FOR NOT BREASTFEEDING

Infants born with galactosemia, a rare inherited disorder, lack the enzyme necessary to break down the sugar found in all milk, including milk-based formulas, other dairy products, and breast milk. These babies must be fed a special lactose-free formula. Newborn screening tests done at discharge from the hospital or birth center detect most cases of galactosemia.

Infants with phenylketonuria (PKU), another rare metabolic disorder, require a diet with little phenylalanine, an amino acid. Because breast milk is low in phenylalanine, a baby with PKU may be breastfed part-time provided she is also fed phenylalanine-free formula. Her blood level of phenylalanine must be monitored to be sure that it remains between 5 and 10 milligrams per deciliter. A pediatric dietitian can help set up a regimen that includes limited breastfeeding.

THE NEAR-TERM BABY

Barring any health complications, babies who are born three to five weeks before the due date are usually treated like any other newborns by physicians and nurses, and parents are encouraged to do the same.

Like full-term infants, near-term infants tend to breathe more regularly, maintain a higher blood-sugar level, and cry much less if allowed to rest unswaddled against the mother's bare chest immediately after birth. If your baby is healthy at birth, you will probably be permitted to hold him skin-to-skin right after he is dried. Your baby may crawl to your breast and latch on to it unaided within the first hour or two of life. Bathing, weighing, and eye treatment can be postponed for an hour or so or until you and your baby are able to complete the first feeding.

It is important to understand, however, that a baby born a few weeks early doesn't behave exactly like a baby born at term. You may find that your baby tends to be extra sleepy and to nurse inconsistently. He may be vigorous at some feedings and inefficient at others. He may fall asleep at the breast before he has taken in sufficient milk. Unless you wake him every two and a half to three hours, he may sleep too long between feedings. He may fail to gain weight; he may even lose weight.

A few days of sluggish nursing and limited milk removal could have a devastating effect on your milk production. To ensure a plentiful supply for a near-term baby, I strongly recommend using a clinical-grade rental pump with a double collection kit. Starting on the third day after birth or earlier, pump each breast for 5 to 10 minutes right after each daytime and evening nursing (freeze the milk you collect for later use). This will help you build an abundant milk supply, which in turn will help the baby get sufficient milk even when he is sleepy at a feeding. See chapter 5 for more information on pumping milk.

When your baby stops sucking during a feeding, compress your breast (see page 37) to increase the flow. This will also help the baby drink more milk.

Watch your baby closely for the signs of adequate milk intake—vigorous sucking and swallowing and frequent stools. Weigh the baby at four to five days of age, and at any time you are concerned about his milk intake, to be sure that he has not lost an excessive amount of weight. (See apendix A.)

If the baby is gaining about an ounce a day or has regained his birth weight at 10 to 12 days, without any supplemental feedings, you can gradually stop pumping over a few days. Weigh the baby once again before returning the pump to the rental station, to be sure he has continued to gain an ounce a day.

If the baby's weight loss nears 10 percent or if he is not gaining at least an ounce a day, offer him the milk you're pumping plus any necessary formula.

A baby born three to five weeks early who is sick may be unable to nurse at first. If this is the case with your baby, you can express your milk for him until he is well enough to begin nursing. In this way he will still benefit from your milk, and you will have established your supply by the time he is ready to begin breastfeeding. For more information, see chapter 5 and the section that follows.

THE VERY PREMATURE OR SICK BABY

When a baby is born sick or very immature—that is, more than five weeks early—the first days after the birth can be overwhelming. In such a case you may have doubts about many things, including your ability to nurse the baby. If your baby is too immature or weak to breastfeed, know that expressing your milk for your baby is very important to his well-being.

Your milk is easier for your baby to digest than formula, and it is particularly suited for a preemie's special growth needs. The fatty acids in human milk promote eye and brain development, which is measurably superior in preterm infants fed mother's milk than in those fed formula. Mother's milk may also reduce a premature baby's risk of developing cerebral palsy. (Lucas, 1992)

Premature infants are at greater risk than full-term infants for developing infections, and preemies are less able to cope with infections when they arise. As you already know, breast milk helps protect a baby against infections. Most protective is the earliest milk, colostrum, which as a preterm mother you'll be making longer than a full-term mother. Doctors think of colostrum as a medicine for preterm babies. As a medicine, colostrum has multiple benefits: It contains a high concentration of antibodies; it creates an environment in the intestinal tract that impairs the growth of harmful bacteria; and it has components that directly attack dangerous germs.

The first drops of colostrum contain the highest concentrations of antibodies, the second drops the next highest, and so on. For this reason, you should number each batch you collect and feed the batches in the sequence in which you have collected them. A nurse or lactation professional can show you how and where to store your colostrum.

KANGAROO CARE

Just as a kangaroo baby, born very undeveloped, is carried and fed in its mother's pouch, a premature human baby benefits from being held next to his parent's body. More and more intensive-care nurseries are allowing and even encouraging parents to practice "kangaroo care": The preemie, dressed only in a diaper and hat, is placed upright between the mother's or father's breasts, inside the parent's shirt or under a blanket. The baby's head is turned to one side, with his ear above the level of the parent's heart.

Premature babies held this way for two hours or more once or twice a day have one-quarter the rate of apnea, or temporary cessation of breathing, of other premature infants. Even a premature baby on a ventilator can be safely moved to the mother without an increase in oxygen. Preemies held kangaroo-style experience no lowering of the heart rate, or bradycardia; in fact, their heart rates are much more stable while they are being held. Their temperatures are stabilized, too, by the warmth of the parent's body. The babies gain weight more rapidly than those kept full-time on a warming bed or in an incubator, perhaps because babies cared for kangaroo-style sleep more deeply, conserving their energy. Faster weight gain means shorter hospital stays; the length of hospitalization for a kangaroo-care baby is reduced by as much as 50 percent. Finally, the skin-to-skin contact not only contributes to parent-baby bonding but also tends to increase the mother's milk production.

Babies who are not yet ready for feedings but are receiving intravenous fluids instead may benefit from having just 0.1 milliliter of colostrum placed in each cheek every three to four hours. This tiny amount will not be swallowed but instead will be absorbed into the baby's lymphatic system to help protect her respiratory and intestinal tracts. If your baby is getting intravenous fluids in place of feedings, be sure to ask if she can have a small amount of colostrum swabbed inside her mouth.

Let the hospital staff know about any medications you take, including any over-the-counter medicines or herbal preparations. Although most medications are safe to take while nursing, a few could harm a sick or premature infant.

If you develop a breast infection (see page 113), you will need to discard any milk you collect, because preterm infants are more susceptible than other babies to bacteria in breast milk.

Refer to chapter 5 for information on expressing milk in general and for a premature or sick baby in particular, and on pumping for longer than a few weeks.

Supplementing Breast Milk. Although breast milk alone is the perfect food for a full-term infant, a preemie, because of her small size and immaturity, may have somewhat different nutritional needs. Many premature infants need supplemental nutrients, especially calcium, phosphorus, and protein. The nurses may mix commercially prepared fortifiers with your milk to provide for these special needs. Usually, the fortifiers are discontinued about the time the baby should have been born. But a preemie needs supplemental iron and vitamins even after discharge from the hospital.

Many premature babies also need a more concentrated source of calories than breast milk. In this situation, a baby may be fed a special preemie formula along with breast milk. A possible option is to feed hindmilk—the fattier milk produced after the first few minutes of pumping (see below). Feeding hindmilk exclusively will speed the weight gain of premature infants.

COLLECTING HINDMILK FOR A PREMATURE OR SICK BABY

Very small premature babies and babies with heart or lung problems may be able to take only small amounts of milk at their feedings. To compensate for smaller feedings, these babies may require higher-calorie milk to grow well. When milk lets down, it starts out as low-calorie *foremilk* and gradually becomes more and more fatty. The milk expressed or fed last contains the most fat. This milk is referred to as *hindmilk*. Feeding hindmilk can be very helpful in achieving good weight gain in a preemie or a baby who has heart or lung problems.

To collect hindmilk separately from foremilk, pump for about 2 minutes after the milk lets down, and then stop pumping and switch collection bottles. Pump again until the breast is completely drained. Label the first bottles as foremilk, the second as hindmilk. Provide the hindmilk for the baby's immediate needs, and freeze the foremilk for the future (for use during separations or for supplementation).

When Breastfeeding Can Begin. The preterm or sick newborn is ready to begin feedings at the breast when his overall condition is stable. It's impossible to know just when a baby will reach this point. If he has poor muscle tone, if he still requires a ventilator, or if he is not yet able to coordinate sucking, swallowing, and breathing, he may not be ready for breastfeeding.

When a baby is ready for oral feeding, breastfeeding is far better for him than bottle-feeding. Studies show that preemies at the breast have better respiratory rates, heart rates, and blood oxygen levels than preemies fed from a bottle. Many doctors tell mothers that breastfeeding is more stressful for preemies than bottle-feeding, but in fact the opposite is true. If there is doubt about the safety of your breastfeeding your preemie, the baby's heart rate and respiration can be observed on the electronic monitor during feedings.

When you begin nursing, try to keep your expectations modest. Preemies' abilities at the breast vary greatly, but most are unable to complete an entire feeding at first.

Have a nurse or lactation consultant help you during the first few sessions. Your goal is to position the baby well for nursing and to encourage her to latch on to the breast. These early practice sessions go best when the baby is awake and alert and the breast is not overly full. Keeping the baby snugly wrapped in a blanket could discourage her interest; it's better to hold her undressed against your skin, with a blanket draped over both of you. The nurse can check the baby's skin temperature after 5 to 10 minutes.

The crossover hold and the football hold (see page 30) are the positions of choice for nursing a premature baby as both of these positions support the baby's head. Place your hand around the baby's head with your fingers behind and below her ears. Support her neck and shoulders with the palm of your hand and your wrist. With your thumb at the point where the baby's nose will touch the breast, compress the breast with your fingers. Lightly stroke the baby's upper lip with your nipple to signal her to open her mouth wide. As soon as she does, pull her head and shoulders toward you so that the nipple is on top of her tongue and far back in her mouth.

While you are nursing your baby, you should eventually be able to hear her swallowing. This means she is sucking effectively and getting your milk. If you do not hear swallowing, make sure the baby is actually latched on to the breast. Her suction should be so strong that it is hard to pull her off. You should not see dimples in her cheeks or hear clicking noises as she sucks. These signs would indicate she was sucking on her tongue and not on your breast. Gently squeeze the breast while the baby is latched to increase the amount of milk the baby receives.

Once latched on to the breast and sucking, a preemie may fall asleep after just a few minutes. Again, preemies' abilities at the breast vary greatly, so be patient. As long as you have positioned your baby correctly and are encouraging her to open her mouth, you have been successful.

If the baby sucks well at the first breast and seems ready for more, you can simply transfer her to the other side without turning her, or you can reposition her in the opposite arm using the football hold.

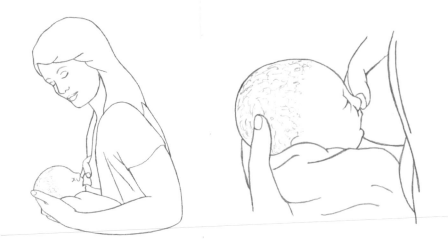

Getting a preemie to latch on requires extra effort: Use the crossover or football hold.

Until she is sucking vigorously at the breast, the baby may need a supplement after nursing. Most hospitals give nursing preemies supplements by bottle; others give them by passing a soft tube through the nose or mouth into the stomach, to avoid "nipple preference." Be sure to pump after feeding sessions and collect your milk so it can be fed to your baby as a supplement. Until your baby is nursing without any supplemental feedings, you will need to continue expressing milk after each nursing to maintain your milk supply.

Difficult Latch-On. Many premature infants have difficulty latching on, due to their immaturity as well as having received rubber nipples as pacifiers or for feedings. Some babies have trouble learning to lower their tongue to latch on, whereas others seem unable to identify their mothers' nipples in their mouths.

Premature infants who are having trouble latching on or drawing milk from the breast may do better with a small-sized nipple shield (see page 58). Nipple shields seem to help immature babies recognize that there is something in their mouths, and this recognition stimulates them to begin sucking. You will want the help of a lactation professional in determining exactly which size shield works best for your nipples and the baby's mouth.

If your baby is unable to latch on to the breast even with a nipple shield, refer to "Difficult Latch-on: Refusal to Nurse," page 57. In my experience, a premature infant typically learns to nurse after a period of daily practice approaching the mother's due date.

THE TRANSITION TO FULL-TIME NURSING

While you and the baby are establishing nursing, you may wonder how much milk the baby is taking. Although mothers and health professionals often try to gauge the baby's milk intake by how long he nurses, how much swallowing can be heard, or whether the baby will take supplemental milk, none of these methods are accurate. The best way to determine the baby's milk intake is to weigh him before and after nursing, in the same diaper and clothing, on an electronic gram scale. Each gram of weight gain equals 1 milliliter of milk intake.

How much breast milk a baby should take at each feeding can be calculated by multiplying the baby's weight in kilograms by 22.5. This will give you in milliliters the amount of milk the baby needs at each of eight daily feedings. For example, if a baby weighs 2.2 kilograms, he will need 49.5, or approximately 50, milliliters of milk each time he nurses, for a total of eight times per day. If the baby takes 30 milliliters during the nursing session, he will need an additional 20 milliliters after nursing to gain an adequate amount of weight.

While you are in the hospital, have your baby weighed on the nursery's scale before and after nursings. If you do this at each nursing, you should begin to develop a sense of how much milk the baby is taking at any feeding. Once at home, you may need weight checks only every two days or so to help you judge how much supplement the baby needs. If you want to continue pre- and post-feeding weight checks at home, rent a highly accurate electronic scale.

NURSING MORE THAN ONE

Needless to say, caring for two or more babies takes a tremendous amount of time and energy. Breastfeeding multiples is not only more healthful and economical than giving them formula, but in many ways it is more convenient. Mothers of twins often say that nursing is easier and less time-consuming than preparing and feeding bottles, particularly when a woman has mastered the skill of nursing two babies at the same time.

Although many mothers worry about being able to produce enough milk for more than one baby, most women are capable of producing plenty of milk for two and even three babies.

As soon as you become aware of the twins during pregnancy, you should begin some special preparations. You will want to arrange for as much help as possible for the first several weeks after the birth. It's also a good idea to get to know other mothers who have successfully nursed their twins. Many communities have organizations for mothers of twins. You might also contact your local breastfeeding support group; such a group usually provides literature on caring for and nursing twins.

Approximately half of all twins are born prematurely. During pregnancy you can do much to lessen the risk of premature delivery and other complications by maintaining a diet high in calories—at least 2,900 a day—and protein—at least 110 grams a day. Talk with your health-care provider about monitoring yourself for signs of preterm labor. Identifying regular contractions, even if they are mild, is important to prevent premature birth.

Establishing an Abundant Milk Supply. Making enough milk for two or more babies depends on the frequent and complete drainage of the breasts. Multiples who are born early or of low birth weight may not consistently nurse effectively enough to stimulate abundant milk production. For this reason I recommend using a clinical-grade rental pump, with a double collection kit, whenever multiples are born three or more weeks before the due date or weigh less than 6 pounds each. See chapter 5 for guidelines on expressing milk for near-term and very preterm infants. Even if your babies are healthy and latching on to the breast frequently, pump for 5 to 10 minutes after each nursing to ensure complete drainage of the breasts and to stimulate abundant milk production. Read "The Near-Term Baby," page 79, for more information on nursing premature babies and chapter 5 for guidelines on expressing milk.

If the babies are in a special-care nursery and are unable to nurse, use the clinical-grade pump at least eight times every 24 hours. Read "The Very Premature or Sick Baby," page 80, and see page 136 for information on expressing milk. You should aim to produce 20 to 24 ounces of milk per day for each of your babies

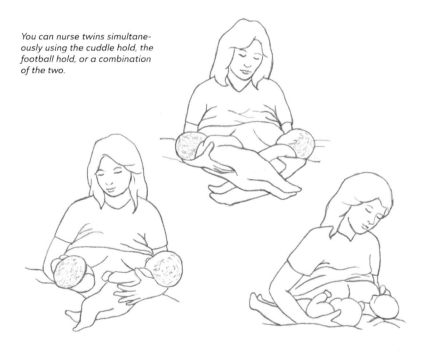

You can nurse twins simultaneously using the cuddle hold, the football hold, or a combination of the two.

Breastfeeding Two or More. You should nurse each of your babies at least eight times in every 24 hours. This may mean waking smaller babies every three hours during the day and evening for feedings, and every four to five hours in the night, until they are gaining weight well without any supplementation.

Some mothers prefer nursing their babies together as much as possible, whereas others choose to nurse them separately. Nursing two at once certainly saves time, and it may be necessary when both of the babies are hungry. If you want to nurse the babies together, there are three basic positions you can try:

- Both babies in the cuddle hold with their legs side by side or crossed over each other
- One baby in the cuddle hold and the other in the football hold
- Both babies in the football hold

During the early weeks, you may need assistance getting the babies on the breast at the same time. You will also probably need a few pillows for positioning. (Special pillows are available for nursing twins.) It may be easier to position the baby who nurses less vigorously first and then put the vigorous nurser to the breast. Nursing the twins simultaneously should get easier as they get older and need less head support and assistance latching on.

Nursing the babies separately, each baby on one breast only, may be easier to manage and will allow you more time with each individually. You may decide to feed each baby whenever she seems hungry, or you may prefer to encourage the babies to eat and sleep on approximately the same schedule. To maintain a similar routine for both babies, simply offer the breast to the second baby, waking her if necessary, after nursing the first. Although most twins eventually develop a preference for one breast over the other, it is wise to alternate the babies at each feeding during the early weeks so the breasts will be evenly stimulated; this is particularly important when one baby is more active than the other. Keeping a simple written record may be helpful at first.

Mothers of triplets generally nurse two babies simultaneously and then the third baby from both breasts, or else another caregiver gives the third baby a bottle. Again, alternate the babies from one feeding to the next.

During the early weeks, if the babies are gaining weight adequately, substituting bottle-feedings for nursings is best avoided. You want to be sure your breasts are stimulated by the babies' sucking so that milk production remains adequate. Forgoing the bottle also helps minimize the occurrence of plugged ducts and breast infections.

Caring for Yourself. For the mother who is nursing two or more babies, getting plenty of rest, food, and drink is essential. Most nursing mothers are naturally more hungry and thirsty than usual. If you take on too much and become fatigued, though, you may lose your appetite and too much weight. Nutritionists recommend that a mother nursing twins consume at least 3,000 calories daily. Your diet should include high-protein foods and a quart or more of milk a day, the equivalent in other dairy products, or a calcium supplement. Vitamin C and B-complex supplements or brewer's yeast may also be beneficial.

THE BABY WITH NOISY BREATHING (LARYNGOMALACIA)

A baby born with this abnormality has "squeaky" breathing. The larynx, or voice box, is malformed, causing the tissues to flop over and partially block the airway opening. The cause of this condition is thought to be congenital, but relaxation of the upper airway or low muscle tone may also be factors. When the baby breathes in, the larynx is partially obstructed, and you hear a high-pitched, squeaky sound known as stridor. This is the most common cause of noisy breathing in infants.

Typically this noise begins during the first two months of life, often in the very first days. Sometimes the sound is confused with nasal congestion, but no nasal discharge is present, and the sound persists. For most infants, laryngomalacia is not serious. Despite having noisy breathing, they are able to eat and grow. The stridor is often more pronounced when the baby is lying on his back or crying, and sometimes during and after feedings. Some infants with laryngomalacia also have problems with reflux (causing spitting up and vomiting), because they have more stomach acid than other babies. The stridor commonly seems to get worse between four and eight months of age, and most babies outgrow it by 18 to 20 months, when the laryngeal structures develop more.

Babies with mild stridor may do better with short, frequent feedings in a more upright or forward-leaning position—that is, with the mother reclined and the baby lying on top.

A small percentage of babies with laryngomalacia do struggle with breathing, eating, and gaining weight. Symptoms that require prompt attention include not breathing for more than 10 seconds, turning blue around the lips, or the baby's chest pulling down, also known as retracting, without relief after being wakened or repositioned. Some babies may choke while feeding or inhale milk into their lungs. Infants with reflux may be given medications that may worsen the laryngomalacia symptoms. If the symptoms are severe, other tests are often done to evaluate the condition. A few infants may require tube feeding or even surgery.

A website devoted to helping parents whose infants have laryngomalacia can be found at www.copingwithlm.org.

THE BABY WITH A BIRTH DEFECT

A baby with a birth defect may need breast milk, and the comfort and security of the breast, even more than other infants. Nursing such a baby is usually possible, but the mother must be supported in her efforts. Although some mothers of babies with birth defects have been discouraged from even attempting breastfeeding, many have gone on to nurse their babies successfully.

Depending on your baby's problem, you may be able to begin nursing right after birth, or you may need to express milk for a while (see page 136). Whatever the circumstances, it may be helpful to seek guidance from a lactation professional.

Heart Defect. Infants with minor heart defects generally have little trouble breastfeeding. The exception is the baby with a severe defect, who may become easily fatigued or stressed during feedings; he will start breathing rapidly, his heart will beat faster, and his overall color may change. His growth may be greatly affected by his heart abnormality. He may also be more prone to infections and therefore in greater need of breast milk than other babies.

A baby who is getting a normal amount of breast milk but is gaining insufficient weight may grow better if he receives extra high-calorie hindmilk. Provided your milk supply is abundant, pump for 2 minutes or so to remove the lower-calorie foremilk, and then nurse the baby. This will provide him with a feeding that is higher in calories.

If your baby becomes stressed during feedings, nurse him more frequently for shorter periods of time. He may also be more comfortable if you hold him upright for nursing, as in the football hold.

Cleft Lip and Palate. The baby born with a cleft lip, palate, or both may have difficulty latching on and sucking effectively, so feeding her may present special challenges. Breastfeeding may be possible, depending on the location and extent of the cleft, but most of these babies, particularly those with cleft palates, are unable to get enough milk from nursing alone. Yet breast milk helps reduce the number and severity of ear and respiratory infections, which are more common in these babies than in others. Many mothers of babies with clefts, therefore, pump their milk and feed it to their babies using whatever method works best for the baby.

The baby born with a cleft lip alone may have little difficulty nursing. Until the lip is repaired, usually when the baby is several weeks old, she may need to be positioned with the cleft sealed, to permit suction. You may be able to create a complete seal just by pulling the baby close against your breast so that your breast occludes the cleft. If you find that your baby has more difficulty nursing on one side than the other, try using the football hold on that side.

Whether a baby with a cleft palate can nurse usually depends on the location and extent of the cleft. When it is in the soft palate only, the baby may or may not be able to nurse without much difficulty. It's best to position her so her head is raised; milk may come out of her nose if you feed her while she is lying flat. Ask the baby's doctor or a lactation professional about devices and techniques to help with feedings. An infant can be fitted with an obturator, a plastic dental appliance that covers the cleft and allows for adequate sucking. Some lactation professionals have reported success with the use of a nursing supplementation device and certain positioning techniques.

If the baby has a cleft palate and is unable to latch or effectively create suction, use a fully automatic electric breast pump every two to three hours around the clock, to stimulate and maintain an abundant milk supply. A clinical-grade rental pump with a double collection kit is most efficient and requires the least amount of pumping time. See chapter 5 for more information on expressing milk.

Bottle-feeding a baby with a cleft lip or palate can also be challenging. The nursing staff should have special feeders of various types that you can try while you are in the hospital. The SpecialNeeds Feeder (formerly called the Haberman Feeder) has worked well for some of my clients.

A cleft palate is generally not repaired until the baby is one to two years old. In the meantime, nursing can be difficult or even impossible. In this case, you will probably need to express milk for some time. Pumping and feeding your milk is far cheaper than feeding formula and may be very helpful in preventing ear infections.

Whether your baby has a cleft lip, a cleft palate, or both, closely monitor her weight to make sure that she is getting enough to eat. If your baby is able to latch on and suck but you're unsure whether she is getting enough milk, weigh her every couple of days, and adjust the amount of supplement as needed to maintain a weight gain of about an ounce a day. Renting an electronic scale for a few weeks may be helpful; you can use the scale before and after nursings to determine how much milk the baby is getting, or simply use it daily to check her weight.

DEVELOPMENTAL AND NEUROLOGICAL PROBLEMS

Babies with Down syndrome, hydrocephalus, spina bifida, cerebral palsy, and other neurological problems benefit greatly from breastfeeding. Because nursing provides frequent physical contact, it may be especially valuable to such a baby's development.

If the baby's sucking ability is affected, teaching him to nurse will require a great deal of patience. You may need guidance from a lactation professional experienced with such problems and also from a physical therapist. In this case, start out using the pump after each nursing to bring in and maintain an abundant milk supply. Once the baby is feeding well and gaining weight at the rate of an ounce per day, you can gradually stop pumping.

If your baby is unable to suck, you may need to feed him with a feeding tube. But some babies may be able to nurse with a nursing supplementation device or to drink your expressed milk from a special bottle like the SpecialNeeds Feeder from Medela.

Down Syndrome. Many infants with Down syndrome are able to nurse. Not only does nursing further their development, it also provides them with much-needed protection from illness, as they are at greater risk than most babies for developing infections.

Some babies with Down syndrome have difficulty learning how to latch on and suck effectively. The baby may have weak muscle tone; he may act sleepy and uninterested in the breast. In this case, rouse him frequently for nursing (see "Sleepy Baby," page 61) and pump after nursings until he is gaining weight as expected.

Typically, the baby with Down syndrome grows slowly. If your baby's suck is weak and inefficient, you may need to pump out the milk he leaves in the breast. Regular pumping will allow you to maintain sufficient milk production and provide the baby extra milk, which you can feed as a supplement after each nursing.

Hydrocephalus and Spina Bifida. These birth defects are usually corrected surgically as soon as possible. Until the baby can begin to nurse, the mother must express milk. For many such babies, positioning at the breast requires special attention so that they are protected and comfortable.

Cerebral Palsy. Babies with cerebral palsy may also be able to nurse, depending on the severity of their condition. Breastfeeding problems that occur are usually related to either (1) poor muscle tone and a weak suck or (2) excessive muscle tone (rigidity and abnormal posture), tongue thrusting, clenching of the jaw, and difficulty swallowing. Both of these situations usually lead to slow weight gain. Some infants with cerebral palsy are able to breastfeed successfully with a nursing supplementation device. A baby with cerebral palsy who struggles with bottle-feeding may do well with a SpecialNeeds Feeder.

THE LEARNING PERIOD:
The First Two Months

AFTER THE FIRST WEEK, you may already be feeling energetic and confident in your abilities as a new mother—or you may be exhausted, overwhelmed, and perhaps troubled by some aspect of breastfeeding. In any case, it is important to realize that the first two months after giving birth are a time for adjustment and learning. Mothers normally have questions and concerns about themselves, their babies, and nursing during this period.

NOW THAT YOUR ARE POSTPARTUM

CARING FOR YOURSELF

Your Nutritional Needs

During the six weeks after birth, all of the many changes of pregnancy are reversed. Virtually every system in your body will go through some readjustment. As your uterus shrinks in size and the inner lining is shed, a new layer is formed. The vaginal flow, or lochia, decreases in amount and progresses to pink or brown and then to white. Many women continue bleeding throughout the first month. Intermittent spotting is common. Too much activity may cause the lochia to become heavier and turn red again—a signal that you should slow down.

If you have had a vaginal birth, your vagina, perineum, urethra, and rectum have undergone considerable stress. Frequent warm baths will speed healing and help relieve discomfort—unless you have hemorrhoids, in which case ice packs may be preferable. Menstrual pads soaked with witch hazel and then frozen are very soothing for hemorrhoids.

Kegel exercises will help this area return to normal by strengthening the entire pelvic floor. These exercises are simple and can be done anytime, anywhere. Several times a day, tightly squeeze the muscles around your anus, then around your vagina and urethra. Gradually work up to 100 "kegels" a day.

If you have had a cesarean birth, keep in mind you are recovering from major abdominal surgery. Most likely, you will need to take pain medication for the first week or so. Using a mild pain reliever such as acetaminophen (Tylenol) or ibuprofen (Motrin, Advil) every few hours may be enough to keep you feeling comfortable. If you are prescribed a narcotic pain reliever, use it only when over-the-counter medications are not enough. Taking a narcotic pain reliever often and for more than one week could make your baby sleepy and could possibly even cause you to have withdrawal symptoms—depression and anxiety, crying, difficulty sleeping, nausea, vomiting, diarrhea, excessive sweating, and dilated pupils—when you stop taking the medication.

You may be bothered by an uncomfortable sensation that your abdominal organs could fall out. A lightweight girdle or a wide band such as the Belly Bandit or the Cinch (available in maternity stores and online) might provide some welcome support.

Constipation is a common complaint in the weeks after giving birth. You can best prevent it by drinking plenty of fluids, eating foods with a lot of fiber, and getting regular exercise. Be aware that some laxatives could affect the baby through your milk, causing cramping, excessive stools, and even weight loss.

Night sweats are very common in the first few days after birth, and they sometimes continue for several weeks.

Starting at approximately six to twelve weeks after birth, some women experience generalized hair loss telogen effluvium. Because of the hormonal changes following birth, hair follicles simultaneously move from the growing phase (which they were in during pregnancy) to the resting phase of their development. Postpartum hair loss is seldom severe, and women never go bald because of it. The period of hair loss lasts three to six months. It has no relationship to breastfeeding.

Most women experience emotional changes during the postpartum period, and some notice problems with mental function, too. Anxiety, moodiness, and irritability are common responses to the hormonal changes that occur after giving birth, as well as to the tremendous responsibility of caring for a new baby. Forgetfulness, inability to concentrate, and difficulty expressing thoughts are also common complaints. All of these problems normally pass with time, good food, plenty of rest, and social support.

Because of the rapid physical changes of the postpartum period and the tremendous amount of time and energy needed to care for and nurse a baby, rest should take high priority for all new mothers. Fatigue can slow recovery from birth and may lead to tension, inability to cope, poor appetite, and depression. Try to take at least one nap every day during these important first weeks. Do essential household chores and activities while the baby is awake so that you can nap together. Tucking the baby in with you at naptime and bedtime may help you both sleep better. Getting plenty of rest now will contribute greatly to your sense of well-being and your breastfeeding success.

After a couple of weeks, some light exercise can do much to renew your energy. A brisk 20-minute walk with the baby can be invigorating; the fresh air will do you both good. Many community centers offer exercise programs for new mothers. Often the babies are included in the exercises, and sometimes infant care is provided. Some people have claimed that exercise causes lactic acid to build up in breast milk, and that this makes babies refuse to nurse, but in fact moderate exercise has little or no effect on the composition or volume of breast milk. With whatever activity you choose, however, you will want to start out slowly.

You may feel isolated as a new mother, especially if you have left work or school—and most of your friends—to care for the baby. You need adult companionship. Check with your childbirth educator or public-health nurse about groups for new mothers. Attending La Leche League meetings, taking a mother-baby exercise class, or socializing with women from your childbirth class are excellent ways of getting out with the baby and getting to know other new mothers.

Drinking Enough. Maintaining an adequate intake of fluids is usually not a problem for the nursing mother. Most women are naturally more thirsty while they are breastfeeding. Contrary to popular belief, forcing fluids beyond satisfying natural thirst does not increase milk production. But when a nursing mother does not drink six to eight glasses of fluids every day, dark, concentrated urine and constipation usually result. You may need to make a conscious effort to increase your fluid intake.

Eating Well. Provided you established good eating habits during pregnancy and gained an adequate amount of weight, you probably won't need to change your diet much at all. Nursing mothers are often told to add about 500 calories, including 65 grams of protein, to their pre-pregnancy diets. Recent research, however, indicates that many mothers may not need this much food, so don't feel you must eat more than you want. You can get extra nutrients in between-meal snacks, perhaps during nursings: Half a sandwich and a glass of milk or a half cup of nuts will supply about 500 calories. Some mothers experience a temporary loss of appetite during the first couple of weeks after delivery. Eating smaller, more frequent meals or snacks may be more appealing than three big meals each day.

You may feel discouraged that your shape is not back to normal. The clothes in your closet may seem as if they belong to someone else. Although you lost some weight when you delivered, you are probably still pounds away from your usual weight. During the early months of breastfeeding, this extra fat is a useful energy store. If you let your appetite guide you as you continue nursing, you will probably lose the excess weight gradually and feel good while doing it. Dieting during the early weeks is not a good idea.

If you prefer to monitor your caloric intake closely, you can estimate your daily caloric needs by multiplying your current weight by 15. Add 500 to your total to meet the caloric needs of nursing (if you are nursing twins, add 1,000 calories).

Example: 135 pounds × 15 = 2,025 calories + 500 calories = 2,525 calories

A moderately active woman can expect to lose a pound every two to three weeks on this caloric intake. If you are very active and have no problem controlling your weight, or if you burn calories slowly, you will need to adjust the figures somewhat: Multiply your weight by 17 (high activity) or 13 (low activity). The minimum safe food intake for a nursing mother of average size is about 1,800 calories per day.

Milk production is largely independent of nutritional intake during the first few months of breastfeeding. This is partly because the fat accumulated in pregnancy is available as a ready supply of calories. When a mother's diet is inadequate, however, milk production usually continues at her expense—leading to fatigue, listlessness, and rapid weight loss. Some women have trouble finding time to fix nutritious meals for themselves when they are at home alone with the baby. If you find yourself in this situation, start the day with a good breakfast, and then snack throughout the day on nutritious foods such as hard-boiled eggs, leftover chicken or beef, cheese, peanut butter, yogurt, seeds, and nuts. Don't forget the fiber: Whole-wheat bread, whole-grain crackers, and raw fruits and vegetables will provide it. Some mothers have developed their own favorite recipes for high-energy blender drinks using ingredients such as milk, yogurt, nuts, and bananas or other fruits.

Low-carbohydrate diets are not recommended while nursing. Whole grains and other high-carbohydrate foods supply nursing mothers with vitamins, minerals, and energy. Low-carbohydrate diets are dehydrating, and they often cause constipation, fatigue, and sleeping problems.

Avoid snacking on foods or drinks that are high in sugar. Refined sugar provides only "empty" calories—empty, that is, of vitamins and minerals. Soda, cookies, and candy will not provide sustaining energy and may diminish your desire for more nutritious foods.

Mothers who are vegetarians can certainly maintain a diet to support their nutritional needs. But since vitamin B12 is found only in foods that come from animals, deficiencies may occur with a vegan diet, which excludes eggs and milk products as well as meat. For vegans, supplementation with up to 4 milligrams of vitamin B12 per day is recommended.

Although most nutritionists recommend that a nursing mother drink three 8-ounce glasses of milk a day, there is no need to drink milk if you don't like it or can't tolerate it. A woman's bone density tends to decrease somewhat during lactation even when her calcium intake is relatively high. This causes no long-term harm. The bones grow denser again after weaning, and some studies suggest that women who breastfeed actually reduce their risk of developing osteoporosis later in life.

SERVING	MILLIGRAMS CALCIUM
yogurt (8 oz.)	288
cheese (1 oz. cheddar or Swiss)	222
cottage cheese (1/2 cup)	110
tofu (1/2 cup)	68
corn tortillas (2)	84

Still, nutritionists recommend that breastfeeding women consume 1,000 milligrams of calcium per day. If you don't drink milk, make sure you're getting enough calcium from other sources, such as those listed in the table above.

Although dark green vegetables in general are rich in calcium (100 milligrams per half cup), the calcium they provide is poorly absorbed by the body. Broccoli is the one exception to this rule. If you do not use dairy products at all, calcium supplements may be necessary. The least expensive supplement, with the highest concentration of calcium, is calcium carbonate. Avoid bone meal, dolomite, and oyster shell, as some types have been found to be contaminated with lead.

Dietary Supplements. If you are well nourished, vitamin supplements are unnecessary while you are nursing, although you may need iron supplements if you are anemic after birth. Also, some nursing mothers develop vitamin B deficiencies, experiencing depression, irritability, impaired concentration, loss of appetite, and tingling or burning feet. A daily B-complex supplement is often prescribed to reverse these symptoms.

Sometimes nursing mothers are advised to take brewer's yeast, a natural source of B vitamins, iron, and protein. Some mothers feel it improves their milk supply or increases their overall energy level. Health-food stores carry brewer's yeast in a powdered form that can be mixed with juice or milk.

If you decide to take vitamin supplements or brewer's yeast, remember that they are no substitute for a varied diet of nutritious foods, and in large quantities they can sometimes be dangerous. There have been reports of fussiness in babies whose mothers take brewer's yeast or large doses of vitamin C. Vitamin B6 supplements in large doses have been reported to reduce milk production.

Foods and Other Substances You May Be Wondering About. There are no foods that should be routinely avoided by nursing mothers, but occasionally a baby will be bothered by something the mother has eaten. Some babies fuss for up to 24 hours after their mothers have eaten garlic, onions, cabbage, broccoli, Brussels sprouts, cauliflower, or chiles. Citrus fruits and their juices, chocolate, and spices such as chili powder, curry powder, and cinnamon can also bother young nursing babies. If your baby has unusual symptoms such as sudden or persistent refusal to nurse, vomiting, diarrhea or green stools, gassiness, redness around the anus, fussiness at the breast, or colic symptoms, see "Concerns about the Baby," page 121.

Caffeine in the mother's diet has been known to cause irritability and colic symptoms in some babies. Caffeine is present in coffee, tea, and many soft drinks. You may want to limit your intake of these beverages.

An occasional glass of wine or beer is not believed to harm a nursing infant. Because alcohol passes through the breast milk, however, moderation is essential.

Mothers who smoke have lower levels of vitamin C in their milk than nonsmokers. Also, secondhand smoke increases a baby's risk of contracting bronchitis, pneumonia, and ear infections and succumbing to sudden infant death syndrome (SIDS). If you smoke, try to limit the amount, and don't do it in your home or anywhere around the baby. Don't let others smoke around the baby, either.

NURSING YOUR BABY

YOUR NURSING STYLE

During the early weeks, each mother develops her own style of nursing. Many women feel comfortable putting their babies to breast whenever the baby signals the desire to nurse. Others expect their babies to fall into a predictable feeding schedule. They may be troubled when their babies nurse irregularly or want to nurse again soon after being fed. These mothers may worry that perhaps they have too little milk or that it is somehow inadequate. Sometimes they feel they must hold the baby off until a certain number of hours have passed since the last feeding. But the breasts do not need to rest for any period of time to build up a supply for the next feeding; they produce milk constantly. The expectation that a baby should nurse on some type of a schedule usually leads to frustration for both mother and baby—and sometimes to breastfeeding failure.

Because breast milk is digested quickly, the newborn infant nurses often—typically between eight and twelve times in a 24-hour period, or about every one to three hours. Not only must a baby nurse frequently to satisfy her hunger and thirst, she also seeks out the breast to satisfy her needs for sucking, security, and comforting. Human infants want to nurse so often that they have been described as continuous feeders.

It is a common misconception that the breast empties in a certain number of minutes, and that a baby should be taken from the breast after those minutes have elapsed. In fact, most mothers experience the release of milk several times during a feeding. The length of time required to complete a feeding varies from baby to baby. The all-business nurser, who swallows continuously with few pauses, may be done in 10 minutes, whereas the dawdler may take up to 40 minutes. The length of nursing time may vary in the same baby from feeding to feeding. Before long, most mothers can tell when their babies have had enough.

Some babies nurse from only one breast at a feeding some or most of the time. This is fine, so long as the baby seems satisfied and is gaining weight adequately. You may prefer to offer only one breast per feeding, in fact, if you have an abundant milk supply. Your baby is more likely to drain the breast completely this way, and complete drainage helps prevent plugged milk ducts and breast infections. Your baby will also be sure to get the rich hindmilk, which is produced in increasing amounts as a feeding progresses.

I strongly recommend that your baby be weighed at 10 to 14 days of age. Although many infants are not scheduled for a routine well-baby exam until three to four weeks of age, a weight check at two weeks can be very beneficial. If the baby is back to her birth weight or beyond, you can be reassured early on that your nursing relationship is pro-gressing well. On the other hand, if the baby has not yet regained her birth weight, you can usually correct this quite easily. When a poor weight gain is not discovered until three or four weeks, it is more likely to upset everyone and may be harder to correct than it would have been at two weeks.

You may find that nursing is the most enjoyable part of your day—a time to sit back, relax, and simply enjoy being with your baby. But it may be difficult at times for you to break away from what you are doing or sit still long enough for the baby to have a leisurely nursing. It may help to make a special little nursing nook for yourself—or two or three nooks in different parts of the house. You might include a book, some magazines, or a notepad within reach. Having the phone nearby may also be handy. Some mothers routinely grab a snack or something to drink just before sitting down to nurse.

Many babies seem to get hungry whenever food is served. To avoid interruptions at dinnertime, you might offer the baby the breast just before preparing your meal. Some parents have found that taking the baby for a walk just before dinner lulls her to sleep so that they can eat without interruption.

YOUR MILK SUPPLY

During these early weeks your milk production may seem somewhat erratic. At times your breasts may feel as if they are bursting with milk. At other times you may worry that there is not enough milk, especially if your breasts seem empty and your baby wants to nurse all the time. Many mothers notice this happening around two to three weeks postpartum and then again at six weeks, when a baby normally experiences appetite spurts and nurses more often to stimulate increased milk production. You can expect fluctuations in your milk supply as production becomes regulated according to the baby's requests.

By six to eight weeks after birth, many mothers notice that their breasts seem smaller or feel less full. This does not usually mean that less milk is being produced, but only that the breasts are adjusting to the large amount of milk within and to the baby's feeding pattern.

Some mothers misinterpret their babies' increased requests and their own softer breasts, and begin offering supplemental bottles. Usually, this marks the beginning of the end of breastfeeding. The mother begins to assume that she cannot make enough milk for her baby, and she offers more and more formula instead of allowing the baby to increase the mother's own supply of milk. After receiving formula, the baby sleeps longer and nurses less often. He becomes increasingly frustrated at the breast as his mother's milk supply dwindles, and breastfeeding is soon over.

Some mothers try to satisfy their babies' hunger with solid foods. But introducing solids during these early weeks is inappropriate, because a young infant is both physiologically and developmentally unable to manage them. His digestive system and kidneys are not mature enough to handle cereals and other baby foods. Because his immune system is still immature, he may develop allergies to solid foods given during this period.

Fluctuations in the fullness of your breasts and in your milk supply will probably pass by the end of the second month after birth. In the meantime, you can be reassured that your milk supply is probably fine if you are nursing at least eight times in each 24-hour period and letting the baby suck for as long as he wants. If you are worried about your milk supply, though, have your baby weighed. A weight gain of at least an ounce a day will tell you that your baby is getting plenty to eat. If you have additional concerns about your milk supply, see "Underfeeding," page 73.

DONATING TO A MILK BANK

While some women are unable to produce sufficient milk, others produce more than their babies can use. Therein lies the beauty of a milk bank, which serves both those in need of milk and those who wish to donate it. If you are considering donating your milk, it is best to wait until your baby is nursing well and gaining weight as expected. Your doctor may even be required to confirm that your baby is thriving before you are permitted to donate. It is also wise to freeze an extra supply of milk for your own baby in the case of an unexpected need, and definitely if you will be returning to work or school. Or you may be a mother who decides to wean and later regrets doing so because your baby is not tolerating infant formula.

Milk banks save babies' lives. The 18 accredited nonprofit milk banks in the United States and Canada help protect the most medically vulnerable infants, who are usually in hospitals. Donors are not paid; rather, the cost of the milk (which is sometimes covered by insurance or by the state) goes to the screening of donors, bacteriologic testing of the milk, pasteurization of the milk, and monitoring a chain of control from the donor to the receiving infant. (There are also for-profit milk banks, like Prolacta, which solicits milk to make a human milk fortifier for premature babies.)

If you are blessed with an abundant milk supply, consider donating some of your milk to a nonprofit milk bank. Like blood banks, milk banks very often experience serious shortages of human milk. Nonprofit banks send milk most often to the sickest babies, whose need for your milk could make the difference between life and death, or serious disability. Visit the Human Milk Banking Association of North America at www.hmbana. org to locate a milk bank site near you. You can be a breast milk heroine!

Casual Milk Sharing

If you are a mother considering accepting milk from a casual milk-sharing organization (such as Eats on Feets or Human Milk 4 Human Babies), keep in mind that someone else's milk may contain toxins, including medications, illegal drugs, tobacco, or alcohol. Certain diseases can be transferred through breast milk as well. Are donor mothers always honest about their intake of tobacco, illegal drugs, and medications? Are all mothers aware of their health history or that of their partners? There is some evidence that this is not always the case. Many milk banks find that donated milk is contaminated with bacteria and must be discarded. Casual peer-to-peer sharing of breast milk could cause harm to a baby receiving milk that has not gone through the process of maternal screening, and culturing and pasteurization of the donated milk. Furthermore, casual milk sharing diverts much-needed milk away from the accredited milk banks, where it can be given to the most medically needy infants.

SCHEDULED FEEDINGS

Some parenting books and classes have promoted a philosophy of scheduled breastfeeding. Called Parent Directed Feeding, the program teaches parents to feed babies on a rigid three- to four-hour schedule and to eliminate nighttime feedings at an early age. The purpose is to relieve parental anxiety and instill a sense of order and discipline in the infant. Although most parents like the idea of predictable, widely spaced nursings and full nights of sleep from the early weeks on, these practices are often associated with low milk production, poor weight gain in the baby, and early weaning. Some babies subjected to this method have become dangerously thin and dehydrated.

Babies do best if they are nursed when they seem hungry. Parent Directed Feeding fails to take into account two important facts about breast milk and breastfeeding. First, nature has designed breast milk to be taken frequently. Low in protein, it is easily and quickly digested. Second, a mother's milk supply depends on frequent, complete drainage of the breasts. If she nurses fewer than seven times in a 24-hour period, her milk production generally declines. Although some mothers can meet their babies' needs with fewer than seven daily feedings, most cannot.

The American Academy of Pediatrics, and every other organization that supports breastfeeding, recommends that babies be fed whenever they show signs of hunger.

INFANT DIETARY SUPPLEMENTS

Supplements sometimes given to nursing babies include vitamin D, iron, and fluoride.
Vitamin D. Known as the "sunshine vitamin," vitamin D is actually a hormone manufactured by the body when the skin is exposed to sunlight. Dietary sources also provide some vitamin D; fatty fish, especially salmon, herring, and tuna, provide high amounts of the vitamin if they are eaten two to three times a week. Some other foods, such as cow's milk, orange juice, and dry cereal, are "fortified" with small amounts of vitamin D.

Vitamin D is important in multiple ways. Because it promotes calcium absorption in the intestinal tract, it is essential for the health of bones. Infants and children who get too little vitamin D are at risk for developing rickets, a painful bone-softening disease that has recently been reported in some American babies. Vitamin D is also a vital part of the immune system and so may make babies less prone to infection. A deficiency of vitamin D is associated with the onset of type 1 diabetes, multiple sclerosis, rheumatoid arthritis, and cancer.

Sunlight, not food additives or supplements, is "the biologically normal and most common way for humans of all ages to develop adequate levels of the hormone 'vitamin D,'" according to Cynthis Good Mojab, a research associate at La Leche League International. The amount of sunlight exposure needed to prevent vitamin D deficiency depends on such factors as latitude, season, altitude, weather, time of day, air pollution, how much skin is exposed, whether sunscreen is applied (since sunscreen prevents vitamin D production), and skin pigmentation. In general, babies achieve adequate vitamin D levels when exposed to sunlight for 30 minutes per week while wearing only a diaper or for two hours per week while fully clothed without a hat. Infants living in northern latitudes may need more sun exposure than this; infants living closer to the equator may need less. Dark-skinned infants may need more sun exposure than light-skinned infants, although researchers have yet to ascertain this. In any case, the exposure must be direct; sunlight that has passed through window glass, Plexiglas, or almost any other plastic does not allow the body to produce vitamin D, because these materials absorb ultraviolet B radiation.

Pediatricians and dermatologists, however, warn parents to keep their babies out of the sun, particularly during the first six months of life. Because sun exposure in infancy has been associated with an increased risk of skin cancer later in life, the American Academy of Pediatrics (AAP) now recommends that all children, including babies who are exclusively breastfed, consume at least 400 IU (international units) of vitamin D per day beginning as soon as possible after birth and continuing through childhood. All infant formulas, like commercially produced cow's milk, are fortified with vitamin D, and babies fed at least 500 milliliters (17.6 ounces) of formula daily get as much vitamin D as the AAP recommends.

But breast milk contains little vitamin D unless the mother takes the vitamin orally in high doses. For exclusively breastfed babies, vitamin D is available in over-the-counter liquid supplements, to be given to the baby by dropper. D-Vi-Sol, made by Enfamil, contains 400 IU of vitamin D per dose; Tri-Vi-Sol, made by the same company, contains vitamins A and C as well as 400 IU of vitamin D. Because breastfed babies don't need supplemental A and C, D-Vi-Sol is generally the better choice between these two. Although the daily dose of each of these preparations is only 1 milliliter, it must be given slowly so that the baby does not gasp, gag, and cough.

Cod liver oil, a supplement much hated by children of generations past, also contains vitamin D as well as vitamin A. The oil is no longer recommended for babies, however, because it can contain mercury and can be toxic at high doses.

There is some controversy about giving oral vitamin D to babies. According to Cynthia Good Mojab, no one has investigated the potential risks, such as aspiration of the liquid, harmful changes in the baby's gut, or increased susceptibility to infection. Since vitamin D is often given in combination with other vitamins, future studies should include the risks of supplementing with those vitamins, too.

An alternative to liquid vitamin-D supplements are the more concentrated Baby Ddrops, which are made by Carlson Laboratories and available at health-food stores and through online pharmacies. One daily drop, providing 400 IU of vitamin D, is placed on the nipple for the baby to take while nursing. The drops are odorless, tasteless, and colorless.

The AAP recommends that a breastfed baby be given supplemental vitamin D until she is weaned to infant formula or, preferably, until she is at least a year old and is drinking at least 2 cups of whole milk per day.

If you want to avoid giving your baby vitamin D supplements, you have a couple of choices. While you're pregnant, you can get plenty of sunshine and dietary vitamin D. This will ensure that your baby is born with enough vitamin D stores to last two months even if she is never exposed to the sun. Then you can postpone giving supplements at least until your baby is two months old.

After your baby is born, you can also take supplemental vitamin D yourself, in the amount of 4,000 to 6,000 IU per day. This will increase the amount of D in your milk enough to protect your baby. The recommended form of supplemental vitamin D is cholecalciferol, or vitamin D3.

Iron. The full-term newborn has sufficient stores of iron for at least the first six months after birth. The small amounts of iron in breast milk are very well utilized by the nursing infant, so iron supplementation is unnecessary. Furthermore, iron supplements can interfere with the anti-infective properties of breast milk.

The baby born prematurely, however, is likely to use up her iron stores earlier than the full-term infant. Supplemental iron is recommended for the premature infant beginning at two months of age or earlier.

Fluoride. This mineral, taken from infancy in water or in supplemental drops, has been shown to reduce childhood dental cavities by 50 to 65 percent. Because little fluoride reaches a baby through breast milk even if the mother drinks fluoridated water, fluoride supplements have sometimes been prescribed for exclusively breastfed babies. Too much fluoride, however, can cause spotting of the developing tooth enamel, and some infants are reported to become fussy and irritable and to have gastrointestinal upsets after being given fluoride. For these reasons, the American Academy of Pediatrics recommends delaying fluoride supplements until a baby is six months old and then using them only if the local drinking water is severely deficient in fluoride, with less than 0.3 parts fluoride per million.

The usual dose of supplemental fluoride is 0.25 milligram per day. Fluoride is available by prescription, either alone or in combination with vitamins A and C, which breastfed babies don't need.

LIFE WITH YOUR BABY

SLEEPING WITH YOUR BABY

Although mothers and babies have slept together at least as long as mammals have roamed the earth, recent warnings about the dangers of bed sharing are worrying new parents. The American Academy of Pediatrics (AAP) has stated that bed sharing can be hazardous under certain conditions, and in 1999 the Consumer Product Safety Commission recommended against parents and babies sleeping together at all. But many physicians, scientists, parents, and sudden infant death syndrome (SIDS) researchers—including one of the Safety Commission members—disagree with this recommendation.

SIDS, or crib death—that is, sleep apnea resulting in a baby's death—has many risk factors. The most common is placing a baby to sleep on her stomach. The second most common is the mother's smoking, either before or after the baby's birth. Formula feeding and overheating are other risk factors, and another is putting the baby to sleep alone in a room. The largest SIDS study to date has shown that infants who sleep alone in a room are more than twice as likely to die from crib death as are infants who share a room with parents. In countries where bed sharing is common, where smoking is not, and where breastfeeding is the norm, SIDS is rare.

Anthropological and developmental studies suggest that mothers and infants are biologically and psychologically designed to sleep next to each other. Parents who sleep with their infants report that they enjoy this closeness and find it makes nighttime parenting easier. Being close to the baby in the night means being more aware of her cues and therefore more responsive to her needs. Even though bed-sharing mothers and babies wake more frequently, they go back to sleep sooner and so get more sleep overall than mothers and babies who sleep separately. Babies who sleep with their parents also cry significantly less than babies who sleep alone.

Because bed-sharing mothers nurse more frequently, they produce more milk than they would otherwise. This can be especially important to women who must spend time apart from their babies during the day. Women who work outside the home also often find that bed sharing helps them feel more connected to their infants.

The AAP recommends that babies sleep in the parents' room for the first six months. James McKenna, an anthropologist at the University of Notre Dame and an expert on infant sleep, also urges parents to sleep in the same room with the baby, if not the same bed, for at least the first six months of life. Dr. McKenna believes that a parent's close breathing may help regulate an infant's own breathing pattern, and that bed sharing may thus reduce instances of SIDS. His review of studies suggests that when a mother and her baby are close enough during nighttime sleep to sense each other in at least two of four ways—sight, scent, sound, and touch—the baby's risk of succumbing to SIDS is significantly decreased. As Dr. McKenna points out, the sharpest recent decline in rates of SIDS and other infant deaths has occurred among middle-class whites, the very group that has most increased its rate of parent-child bed sharing over the same period.

In his sleep laboratory at Notre Dame, Dr. McKenna has found that bed-sharing mothers and their infants are extremely sensitive to each other's movements and physical condition throughout the night, across all sleep stages. For instance, healthy, full-term babies whose air passages become blocked alert their bed-sharing mothers and, under normal circumstances, maneuver out of danger. Babies who sleep alone, Dr. McKenna has found, spend more time in deeper stages of sleep, which may be harmful for babies with inherent arousal deficiencies.

Other researchers have suggested that babies who sleep with their mothers develop into children who are independent, sociable, confident, and well able to handle stress. Children who have never slept in their parents' beds are, according to their parents, harder to control, less happy, more prone to tantrums, more fearful, and more dependent.

There are certainly hazards to avoid in bed sharing, but there are hazards in laying the baby to sleep anywhere. Wherever the baby sleeps, the dangers are mostly the same: pillows, toys, and quilts that could suffocate; cords and ties that could strangle; gaps in which a baby could become wedged; heights from which she could fall; and overheating. Bed sharing poses the additional risk of "overlying"—accidental smothering—but this is generally a concern only when other children are sleeping in the same bed or a parent is intoxicated or extremely exhausted. Generally, adults have a sense of their own boundaries even when asleep; this is why you don't fall out of bed.

If you smoked during pregnancy or if your baby isn't exclusively breastfed, room sharing, rather than bed sharing, may be the safest sleeping situation for your baby, studies show. The reasons for this are unclear.

For most of the benefits of bed sharing with no risk of overlying, you might try placing your baby's bed very close to your own. You can even buy a baby bed that attaches to an adult bed so you can reach your baby without getting up even though she is sleeping on a separate surface. Or you can put your baby in a small bed on top of your own. (See the Snuggle Nest at www.babydelight.com.)

Following are some guidelines for safe infant sleep, with the parents or in a separate bed:

- Use a firm mattress that fits the bed or crib frame well, without gaps in which a baby could become wedged.
- Stretch the sheet tightly around the mattress.
- Avoid nightclothes with strings or ties, both for the baby and, if you're sharing the bed, for yourself and your partner.
- Keep the baby's face uncovered.
- Leave off the comforters, feather beds, stuffed animals, lamb skins, and other soft things that could pose a risk of suffocation. The baby doesn't need a pillow.
- Put the baby on her back or side to sleep.
- Don't smoke, and don't let other people smoke in the house.
- Avoid overheating the room in which the baby sleeps, and avoid overdressing the baby. Keep the room cool if you share a bed so that the warmth of your body combined with the warmth of the covers does not overheat the baby, or have the baby sleep outside the covers.

- Avoid laying the baby to sleep near dangling cords or sashes.
- Don't leave a young baby, especially one born prematurely, to sleep in a car seat or infant seat. If the baby's upper body is inadequately supported, her airway may become blocked.

If your baby sleeps in a crib, follow these guidelines:
- Make sure the rails are no farther than 23/8 inches apart.
- If you use crib bumpers, make sure that they have at least six ties. The ties should be no longer than 6 inches long.
- When the baby learns to sit, lower the mattress so that she can't fall out or climb over the side rail.
- Hang any crib mobile well out of the baby's reach, and remove it when the baby starts to sit or reaches five months of age, whichever comes first.
- When she learns to stand, set the mattress at its lowest level and remove any crib bumpers.
- When she reaches a height of 35 inches or the side rail is less than three-quarters of her height, move her to another bed.
- Remove any "crib gym" when a baby can get up on all fours.
- Dress the baby in a blanket sleeper instead of using a blanket. If you do use a blanket, make sure the baby's head remains uncovered.
- Consider using a baby monitor with the speaker turned toward the baby during naps. Background noise from the monitor may protect the baby as well as bed sharing.

If your baby sleeps with you, follow these guidelines:
- Don't place the bed against the wall or against other furniture, since the baby could become trapped in between.
- If your bed has head- or footboard railings, they should be spaced no wider than 23/8 inches apart.
- Don't leave the baby to sleep alone in your bed.
- Fasten back your hair, if it is very long.
- After drinking or taking drugs that may cause you to sleep too soundly, and at any time that you are extremely exhausted, put the baby to sleep in a separate bed.
- Don't use bed rails in the baby's first year, since she could become wedged between the mattress and the rail.
- Don't let an older sibling share a bed with an infant younger than one year old.
- Don't share a waterbed with your baby, since the surface could hamper breathing if your baby were to turn face down.
- Consider bed sharing carefully if you or your partner is obese. Your weight might create a depression in the mattress that the baby could roll into. Sleeping on a very firm mattress might be safer in this case.
- Don't sleep with the baby on a sofa or overstuffed chair.

Different sleeping arrangements may work best for you at different times. You might place your baby in a bassinet at bedtime but move her into your bed later for night feedings. You might instead nurse the baby to sleep in your bed and then move her to her own bed afterward. Or you might put the baby to sleep in the nursery but then sometimes end up sleeping there all night yourself. You might follow a certain pattern for many months or change more often as your baby grows and your own needs change.

The Nursing Mother's Companion, 7th ed. (see "Suggested Supplemental Reading," page 182) has more detailed guidelines for safe infant sleep.

ILLNESSES: YOURS AND THE BABY'S

When you come down with a minor illness such as a cold or flu, you need not interrupt breastfeeding. Most likely your baby will have already been exposed to the virus that caused you to get sick. In fact, the antibodies you produce against the illness will reach the baby through the milk and may protect him from getting the same sickness. Even though you may not feel much like eating, try to drink extra fluids to keep from getting dehydrated. Should you need to take a medication, even an over-the-counter drug, be sure to check on its safety for the baby. Some over-the-counter cold remedies contain pseudoephedrine, which can decrease milk production, sometimes permanently.

Temporary weaning is also unnecessary if you suspect you have a case of food poisoning, provided your only symptoms are vomiting, diarrhea, or both.

Your milk supply may seem low during or just after an illness, but a few days of frequent nursing will usually bring milk production back to normal.

Should you require hospitalization or surgery, you can continue breastfeeding. If you know ahead of time that you'll need a hospital stay, you can pump and save milk for any time that you may be unavailable to your baby. You may be able to arrange to have your baby stay with you, although the hospital will probably require that another adult be there to care for the baby. Ask if the hospital has a fully automatic breast pump for you to use when you cannot nurse; if not, arrange to bring one along, with a double-pump kit. The hospital may even have a lactation professional on staff who can assist with any breastfeeding problems that arise during your hospitalization.

You won't need to express and throw out milk contaminated by an anesthetic or pain medication. By the time you awaken from anesthesia, there will not be enough of the drug in your body to be a problem for your baby. Pain medications are also safeWhen you are not able to nurse your baby, express your milk every two to three hours during the day and evening and as often during the night as you usually feed the baby. Ask the nurses to wake you as often as you need to pump. They should be able to refrigerate your milk in clean containers that you can take home to your baby.

Should your baby become ill, nursing should certainly continue. Breast milk is the best source of fluids and nourishment for recovery and nursing the best source of comfort. But be aware that sickness often changes a baby's nursing pattern. He may nurse more than usual, or he may lose interest in nursing. Ear infections, sore throats, and fever blisters may make nursing painful for the baby. As long as he is nursing infrequently or is refusing to nurse, be sure to express your milk every couple of hours to keep up your supply.

Colds and stuffy noses can make nursing difficult for a baby. Holding your baby upright while feeding, using a humidifier in the room, or administering saline nose drops and cleaning out his nose may make nursing more comfortable for him. Try the Nose-Frida, a safe, gentle nasal aspirator that captures the baby's nasal discharge and prevents it from contaminating the device, unlike a traditional bulb aspirator. The NoseFrida is available at many stores and online.

Fever is a sign of infection. During the first four months, a temperature above 99°F if taken in the armpit, or 101°F if taken rectally, should be reported to the baby's doctor. If, besides having an elevated temperature, the baby doesn't act like his usual self or he nurses poorly, he should be checked by the doctor. The severity of a fever does not always correspond with the seriousness of an illness; a high fever may appear with a minor infection, and a low fever may accompany a serious infection. Because a fever may lead to dehydration, frequent nursing is very important.

Diarrhea in the breastfed baby, although less common and usually less severe than in the formula-fed baby, is characterized by frequent (12 or more per day), extremely loose or watery bowel movements. Often the stools are foul smelling, and they may contain mucus or blood. Since babies lose a great deal of fluid with diarrhea, they can easily become dehydrated, so frequent nursing is important. With its high water content, breast milk helps replace the lost fluids. Diarrhea generally improves within three to five days. Fever, infrequent feedings, or signs of dehydration (dry mouth, few wet diapers, listlessness) are reasons to notify your doctor. In cases of severe diarrhea, doctors occasionally recommend supplements of an electrolyte solution, such as Pedialyte, in conjunction with nursing.

THE FIRST TWO MONTHS: WHAT'S NORMAL?

During the first two months you can expect your baby will nurse between eight and twelve times a day, including at least once at night. If your baby sleeps four to six hours at a stretch at night or takes a three- to four-hour nap during the day, she will probably want to nurse often during the next few hours to make up for the meal she missed. The baby who is nursing fewer than eight times in a 24-hour period or who is sleeping longer than six hours at a stretch at night is typically the infant who fails to gain enough weight during the early weeks of nursing.

Generally, eight or more wet diapers a day are a sign that the baby is getting enough milk. By two weeks, most nursing infants have regained their birth weight. A gain of at least an ounce a day is normal.

The breastfed baby typically has very loose and seedy-looking stools. During the first month most infants have at least one bowel movement daily. After the first month it is not uncommon for a baby to go several days without a bowel movement. As long as the baby seems comfortable, there is probably no need for concern; your baby is unlikely to be constipated or underfed. The baby who is not getting enough to eat typically has small, and usually infrequent, brown or greenish stools and is gaining less than an ounce a day.

Many mothers continue to experience dripping or spraying milk during or between nursings. But some women stop leaking altogether after the first several weeks, and most gradually notice less leakage.

At some point during the first two months you will probably start to experience the sensations of milk let-down. You may notice this tingling, pins-and-needles feeling in your breasts just before or during a feeding or at any time your baby signals you with his cry.

Occasionally babies spit up after a feeding. Some babies spit up after every nursing. This is usually due to an immature digestive system; what comes up is normally just a few teaspoons. If your baby spits up more, the cause may be certain foods or beverages in your diet (see "Spitting Up and Vomiting," page 121, and "Fussiness, Colic, and Reflux," page 123). In any case, spitting up passes with time; until it does, keep a diaper or small towel handy.

A baby cries for any of a number of reasons. She may be hungry or tired, or she may just want to suck and be held. Sucking at the breast is soothing and comforting for her. Babies usually have a fussy period in the evening. Although many theories have been suggested to explain why this is, most babies are comforted by extra nursing. Try not to assume your milk is somehow lacking. Many mothers who interpret their babies' cries this way begin supplementing with formula and soon find the babies weaned. See "Fussiness, Colic, and Reflux," page 123, for more on why babies cry and how to cope with crying.

During the appetite spurts at about two to three weeks and six weeks of age, your baby may act more fussy than usual and want to nurse more often. After a few days of frequent nursing, your milk supply will increase to meet her needs and she will return to her usual nursing pattern.

Some babies cry hard, as if in pain, for prolonged periods every day. They are said to have *colic*, which is just a name for extreme irritability that continues day after day—for any of a number of reasons. Some cry at the breast or refuse nursing entirely. If your baby has colic symptoms, see "Fussiness, Colic, and Reflux," page 123.

You may have heard that tending to your baby each time she cries will spoil her or will reinforce her behavior and cause her to cry more often. Nothing could be further from the truth. Babies do not cry to exercise their lungs, but because they are in need of something. If your baby's needs are met in infancy, she will develop a sense of security, and she will grow to trust in you and others as well.

During these early weeks, while you are learning about your baby, caring for her needs, and learning to breastfeed, you are apt to experience some feelings of concern, confusion, and perhaps even inadequacy regarding your mothering abilities. Motherhood and breastfeeding may not be exactly what you expected. Your baby's crying and the unpredictability of her sleeping and wakeful periods may be upsetting. The baby's nursing schedule (or lack thereof) and her many needs may make it impossible to feel organized or productive. Perhaps you are disappointed by the lack of help from your health-care providers. Early motherhood may also bring feelings of loneliness and isolation.

It is normal to have mixed feelings about nursing. Try to keep in mind that new motherhood brings a period of uncertainty and adjustment, and that nursing, like mothering, gets easier with time.

The First Two Months

CONCERNS ABOUT YOURSELF

- Sore Nipples
- Breast Pain
- Plugged Ducts
- Breast Infection (Mastitis)
- Breast Abscess
- Breast Lumps
- Leaking Milk
- Overabundant Milk
- Lopsided Breasts
- Nausea or Headache
- Depression and Anxiety
- Dysphoric Milk Ejection Reflex (Bad Feelings While Nursing)

CONCERNS ABOUT THE BABY

- Spitting Up and Vomiting
- Pulling Away from the Breast
- Refusal to Nurse
- Fussiness, Colic, and Reflux
- Underfeeding

CONCERNS ABOUT YOURSELF

Sore Nipples

It can certainly be discouraging when sore nipples persist beyond the first week. If this happens to you, review the information on sore nipples in "Survival Guide: THe First Week." It may be helpful to have your partner or a friend observe your latch-on technique and compare it with the descriptions of latch-on in "Positioning at the Breast," page 29. Babies who are tongue-tied may also cause painful nipples (see page 66). But don't discount the possibility that your nipples are irritated due to thrush or another dermatologic condition.

Thrush nipples. If your nipples suddenly become sore after a period of comfortable nursing, thrush is the most likely cause. This problem occurs when a yeast (monilia) infection in the baby's mouth spreads to the mother's nipples. The nipples become shiny, reddened, swollen, tender, and sometimes cracked. Occasionally, peeling or a red, dotty rash can be seen on the nipples. Some mothers complain of itching; others complain of burning. Thrush sometimes begins after the mother has taken a course of antibiotics or when she has had a vaginal yeast infection (symptomatic or not).

If you suspect a case of thrush, carefully inspect the baby's mouth. You may see white patches on the inside of the cheeks, inside the lips, and possibly on the tongue. Sometimes a baby will have no symptoms in the mouth but will have a diaper rash caused by yeast. A yeast rash often resembles a mild burn; it may be scaly and peeling. It is usually well defined, very red, and a bit raised, but sometimes it looks like just a patch of red dots.

It usually appears in the genital area but may also be noticeable in the folds of the baby's diaper area. A yeast rash will not respond to typical remedies like frequent cleaning and the usual diaper rash creams. For treatment, see page 125.

TREATMENT MEASURES FOR THRUSH NIPPLES

1. The treatment baby doctors usually recommend for thrush is 1 milliliter nystatin suspension (Mycostatin) by dropper into the baby's mouth after every other nursing, or four times daily, for 14 days. Wait a few minutes after nursing before giving this prescription medication so it won't be washed out of the baby's mouth by the milk. Half the dose should be dropped into each side of the mouth. Even if the symptoms are gone after a few days, continue the treatment for the full 14 days.

2. To prevent reinfection, the nipples must be treated at the same time as the baby's mouth. The best remedy is nystatin cream or ointment, which, like nystatin suspension, is available by prescription only. (The oral medication can be applied to the nipples instead, but it is usually ineffective.) Your baby's doctor may prescribe nystatin cream for your nipples (and for your baby's diaper rash, if present); if not, call your own doctor for a prescription, or use an over-the-counter antifungal cream such as Lotrimin AF, Micatin, or Monistat 7. Apply the medication after each nursing. Some lactation professionals recommend rinsing the nipples, for the first few days of treatment, with water or a mild solution of vinegar (1 tablespoon vinegar to 1 cup water) before applying the medication.

3. Because nystatin inhibits yeast growth for only about two hours after you swab the baby's mouth, it is often ineffective when used as prescribed. If your baby's mouth isn't clear of thrush after five to six days of treatment, ask your doctor about more frequent dosing, or try using gentian violet, as described in step 4, instead.

4. A 1 percent solution of gentian violet can be purchased without a prescription at most but not all drugstores, so call around before making the trip, or have the pharmacy order it for you. If you can find only 2 percent gentian violet, you can have the pharmacist dilute the solution, or you can do it yourself by placing a few drops in the cap and adding an equal amount of water. Thoroughly swab the affected areas in the baby's mouth using a cotton-tipped applicator, once or twice a day for three days. The solution will stain the baby's mouth purple; take care in applying it so that nothing else turns purple. Some lactation professionals recommend painting the mother's nipples with gentian violet, too, but I don't recommend this treatment if the nipples are tender.

5. Canadian pediatrician and breastfeeding specialist Dr. Jack Newman recommends using grapefruit seed extract (available at most health-food stores) as a nipple solution. Mix five to ten drops of the liquid into 1 ounce of water and rub some of this solution on the nipples and areolas after nursings. The concentration of the grapefruit seed extract can be increased gradually to up to 25 drops in 1 ounce of water. You can use this solution in addition to any topical antifungal cream by alternating it with the cream. If you find that your nipples begin flaking, stop using this solution.

6. If the weather allows, briefly expose your nipples to the sun two or three times daily to hasten healing.

7. Sanitize your breastfeeding supplies to prevent reinfection. If you're using nursing pads, change them at each feeding. If you are using a pump, wash all the parts thoroughly after each use. Bottle nipples, plastic breast shells, and pump parts that come in contact with the breast or the milk should be boiled in water for 5 minutes daily. If your baby uses a pacifier, make sure you boil it daily as well.

8. If thrush and accompanying sore nipples aren't cured by the usual treatment measures, some mothers try fluconazole (Diflucan), an oral antifungal agent. The usual dosage is 400 milligrams on the first day followed by 100 milligrams for the next 13 days. This medication is very expensive, though, and I find that most mothers can overcome yeast infections by using antifungal cream on the nipples and treating the baby's mouth. If you try a course of fluconazole and still suffer with nipple soreness, yeast is probably not the problem.

9. If after the treatment just described your baby shows no signs of thrush but your nipples are still irritated, see a dermatologist. In the absence of visible thrush, pink, burning nipples may indicate nipple dermatitis.

Nipple dermatitis. If you experience pink, tender nipples beyond the first week of nursing and your baby shows no signs of thrush, you may have another dermatologic condition. A dermatologist can probably both uncover the cause of the soreness and offer effective treatment. Before seeing a dermatologist, though, you might ask your regular physician to prescribe Dr. Jack Newman's all-purpose nipple ointment, or APNO. A topical medication that must be specially made up in a pharmacy, APNO includes 2 percent mupirocin ointment (15 grams), an antibacterial; 0.1 percent betamethasone ointment (15 grams), an anti-inflammatory; and 2 percent miconazole or clotrimazole powder, an antifungal. An optional fourth ingredient, ibuprofen, is helpful for pain relief. The ointment is applied sparingly after nursings or pumpings until the nipples are free of pain for a few days, and then gradually used less often.

If your nipples are still tender after treatment with APNO or an antibacterial ointment, I highly recommend seeing a dermatologist.

Painful, blanched nipples. Some women notice that their nipples become painful and pale at the end of nursing sessions. Often this pain and blanching results from poor positioning of the baby at the breast. The compression of the nipples probably causes a vasospasm—a spasm in the blood vessels—which prevents blood from getting to the nipples. You may be able to solve this problem by correcting your latch-on technique (review "Positioning at the Breast," page 29) and by applying warm compresses to the nipples right after nursing.

Sometimes vasospasm in the nipples results from Raynaud's disease or Raynaud's phenomenon (these two are different; the less common Raynaud's disease occurs on its own, whereas Raynaud's phenomenon is associated with illness such as rheumatoid arthritis or repetitive trauma or injury and affects some 22 percent of 21- to 51-year-old women). In both conditions, blood-vessel spasms brought on by a drop in temperature prevent blood from getting to a particular area of the body. Most commonly, Raynaud's occurs in the fingers, typically when a person goes outdoors from a warm building on a cool day. In this case, the fingers turn white and the tips hurt.

When Raynaud's affects the nipples, it causes nipple blanching just after a feeding, probably because the ambient air is cooler than the inside of the baby's mouth. When the baby comes off the breast, the nipple is its usual color, but it very quickly turns white. This blanching is accompanied by burning pain. Then the nipple turns blue; this is caused by deoxygenation of the blood. As the blood starts flowing back to the nipple, the nipple returns to its normal color, and the mother may experience a throbbing pain. The three-phase color change—from white to blue to red—suggests a diagnosis of Raynaud's phenomenon rather than poor positioning. The nipple colors and the types of pain may alternate for several minutes or as long as an hour or more.

If you have Raynaud's phenomenon, avoiding cold is important. Your entire body needs to be kept warm. Breastfeed in a warm place, wear warm clothing, and avoid exposure to cold at all times. If you experience a painful vasospasm, applying warm, moist cloths to your nipples may help. Avoid smoking and caffeine.

Dietary supplements may help alleviate vasospasms caused by Raynaud's phenomenon. Some women have used a combination of calcium (2,000 milligrams per day) and magnesium (1,000 milligrams per day). So far, however, no studies have tested the effectiveness of this remedy. Jack Newman, a pediatrician, reports that vitamin B6 often helps with Raynaud's phenomenon and is safe to use. He suggests a dosage of 150 to 200 milligrams once a day for four days. If the symptoms don't lessen in this much time, vitamin B6 probably won't help at all, Newman says. But if the pain resolves, he suggests taking a reduced dose of 25 milligrams once a day until you are pain-free for a few weeks. If the pain returns with the smaller dose, you can return to the higher dose (Newman and Pitman, 2006).

Various drugs have been investigated for the treatment of Raynaud's phenomenon. The most effective among them is nifedipine, which is primarily used to treat hypertension. Nifedipine is probably safe to use, since very little of the drug (less than 5 percent of the total dose) appears in the breast milk, and side effects in the mother are uncommon (the most frequent side effect is a headache). The usual dosage of nifedipine is one 30-milligram slow-release tablet per day for two weeks. If the nipple pain returns, as it does in about 10 percent of mothers, a second course can be taken. Women rarely require more than three courses.

Breast Pain

For a variety of reasons, your breasts may begin to hurt during nursing or become perpetually tender or sore. If this happens, it is important to identify the cause so that you can take any necessary action.

Uncomfortable engorgement can occur any time the breasts become overly full—when the baby misses a feeding, for example, or when he begins to sleep longer at night (see "Engorged Breasts," page 47).

Most mothers begin noticing normal let-down sensations during these early weeks. Let-down may be experienced as a mild ache at the start of nursing or a tingling, pins-and-needles sensation.

A deep pain, often described as "shooting," that occurs just after nursing is thought to be related to the sudden refilling of the breast. These pains disappear after the first few weeks of nursing. Blocked nipple pores can also cause stabbing pains (see below).

Pain during nursing, often described as burning or stinging, is usually associated with thrush. The nipples may be pinker than usual. Sometimes a rash may be visible. See "Thrush Nipples," page 108, for additional information on causes and treatment.

If you can feel a tender area or painful lump in your breast, see the following section.

Plugged Ducts

You may experience a plugged milk duct as a small, tender spot or as a large area of the breast that feels overly full and does not soften with nursing. If you look in a mirror, the skin over the area may appear reddened.

Occasionally a plug in one of the nipple openings blocks the milk flow and causes a backup of milk in the breast. If the nipple looks normal in color but you can see a white pimple (a "bleb") on the end of the nipple, particularly right after the baby comes off the breast, the problem may be a plugged nipple pore. Plugged nipple pores are often associated with stabbing breast pain, especially right after nursing.

Plugged ducts are most common during the early weeks of nursing, but they can occur at any time during breastfeeding. They occur for various reasons. In the early weeks and months, they frequently seem to be caused by incomplete drainage of the breast. Mothers with high milk production, including those nursing twins, tend to be more prone to plugged ducts. Interrupting the baby's nursing to switch to the other breast before the baby signals that he is finished may lead to a plugged duct. A plugged duct may follow a missed feeding or a long stretch at night without nursing. Overly tight bras, especially underwire types, may obstruct milk flow and lead to plugged ducts. Baby carriers with tight straps can also cause this to happen.

For unknown reasons, plugged ducts seem to be more common during the winter months. Some breastfeeding specialists feel that mothers who drink an insufficient amount of fluids, who become slightly dehydrated due to a cold or flu, or who are overly fatigued may also be more susceptible to developing plugged milk ducts.

Any breast lump that does not get significantly smaller within a week should be examined by a doctor.

TREATMENT MEASURES FOR PLUGGED DUCTS

1. Remove your bra if there is any question that it may be too tight or may be pressing into part of your breast.
2. Before nursing, apply moist heat to the breast for 15 to 20 minutes.
3. Nurse frequently, at least every two hours. Begin each nursing on the affected breast.

4. While nursing, gently massage the breast just behind the sore area.

5. If you are following the preceding recommendations but notice no change in your breast after a feeding or two, try positioning the baby with his chin close to the plugged duct, if possible, to promote better drainage. If this doesn't work, get into the shower. With your breast well soaped, apply steady but gentle pressure behind the plugged area, pressing toward the nipple.

6. Increase your fluid intake so that you urinate more frequently.

7. If the blockage seems to be in the nipple, look for dried milk secretions or a clogged nipple pore, which may resemble a whitehead. If necessary, you can gently remove a visible plug from a nipple opening with a sterilized needle. (Wash your hands well. To sterilize a needle, place the needle in a cup of rubbing alcohol or hydrogen peroxide, and leave it there for 30 seconds. Wash your hands again, and then pick up the needle by the blunt end.) Using the needle to open the "bleb" may cause a little bleeding, but you probably won't feel any pain.

8. If nursing is too painful or if you suspect the baby isn't draining the affected breast well, begin pumping your breasts after or instead of nursing. Renting a clinical-grade pump for a couple of days may be best. If you are pumping instead of nursing, pump very often. Some mothers have found that using Pumpin' Pal Super Shields while pumping can clear up a plugged milk duct (see page 112). Occasionally a mother who pumps with a plugged duct will get pink milk from a bit of blood coming from the plug opening up. There is no need to be alarmed, but avoid feeding that milk to your baby, as blood is a gastric irritant and can cause her to vomit.

9. Be alert for signs of a developing breast infection—fever, chills, and achiness—so you can treat it promptly. (See the section that follows.)

If a plug does not resolve after a few feedings with the above measures, some lactation professionals suggest using an old-fashioned treatment for swelling: Apply castor oil to a warm, moist washcloth, lay it over the sore area, and place a heating pad over the washcloth. Keep the compress and heating pad in place for about 20 minutes before nursing or pumping. This can be repeated before each feeding.

Breast Infection (Mastitis)

Up to 30 percent of all nursing women develop mastitis, or infection of the breast. It occurs most often in the first three months after birth and, interestingly, it is more common during the winter months.

A breast infection is caused by bacteria, often the same ones normally present on the nipples and in the baby's mouth. A breast infection often follows an untreated cracked nipple or a plugged milk duct. It is more likely to occur when the baby (or a pump) is ineffective at draining the breasts. Other possible causes include poor-fitting bras, skipped feedings, infrequent changing of wet breast pads, anemia, stress, and fatigue.

Since mastitis causes flu-like symptoms, women sometimes mistake it for the flu. Headache, general achiness, and a reddened area of the breast are the early symptoms; they are usually followed by fever (typically over 101°F), chills, and weakness. Usually only one breast is affected; it becomes quite tender in the infected area.

Women who promptly apply moist heat to the breast and work on getting it as empty as possible may recover quickly without antibiotics, usually in two days. In one study of women with mastitis, half used no antibiotics, and none of them suffered complications (Riordan and Nichols, 1990). I have come to believe, however, that prompt treatment with antibiotics is indicated whenever a nursing mother has flu-like symptoms and a reddened breast, especially if she has a fever. Some women have permanently lost their milk production from the affected breast following a breast infection, although this has usually occurred when treatment has been delayed. Late treatment can also result in an abscess, which may require surgical drainage. This risk may be greater if you are anemic.

Effective treatment with an antibiotic requires the right choice of antibiotic. The bacterium involved in mastitis is usually *Staphylococcus aureus,* or "staph," which is resistant to amoxicillin, penicillins G and V, and many other antibiotics.

Usually, the most effective antibiotics against this organism are cloxacillin and dicloxacillin, and cephalosporins, such as cephalexin (Keflex). Another frequently prescribed penicillin is Augmentin, a more potent form of amoxicillin. Erythromycin, clarithromycin, azithromycin, and clindamycin are used in women who are allergic to penicillin. All of these antibiotics are safe to take while breastfeeding unless the baby is allergic to them (the allergy usually causes a rash).

Recently, some staph infections have become resistant to all penicillins, so if you are not markedly better in three or four days, contact your health-care provider. You may need a different antibiotic, such as clindamycin, co-trimoxazole (Septra), or doxycycline. Mothers who fail to respond to antibiotics may have contracted MRSA, or methicillin-resistant *Staphylococcus aureus.* This bacteria has been cultured in the milk of some mothers who do not seem to be responding to the antibiotics normally used to treat mastitis. If you are still sick after a few days, speak with your doctor about this possibility.

In general, antibiotic treatment for mastitis should continue for 10 to 14 days. It is important to take the antibiotic until it is used up, even if you feel better, because you could develop a resistant infection if you stop too soon.

With prompt and proper treatment the symptoms usually subside within 48 hours. Nurse frequently during this period; discontinuing nursing would slow healing and might lead to the development of a breast abscess. Unless you are expressing milk for a premature or sick baby who is hospitalized, you don't need to worry that the baby will get ill, since the infection involves only the breast tissue, not the milk. Try to identify the probable cause of the infection so you can prevent a recurrence in the future.

Mastitis in both breasts, though rare, can be a sign of B-streptococcal infection, which is transmitted by the infant to the breasts. When both breasts are affected, the baby's doctor should be promptly notified so that the baby can be tested and treated, if necessary.

TREATMENT MEASURES FOR MASTITIS

1. Go to bed, if you haven't already.
2. Remove your bra if you are more comfortable without it or if there is any question that it may be pressing into part of your breast.
3. Nurse frequently, at least every two hours, and begin each nursing on the affected breast. Giving up nursing could slow healing and lead to a breast abscess.
4. If nursing is too painful or if you suspect the baby isn't draining the affected breast well, begin pumping your breasts after or instead of nursing. Renting a clinical-grade pump for a couple of days may be best (see page 140 for advice on expressing milk). If you are pumping instead of nursing, pump very often.
5. Call your doctor, who will probably prescribe antibiotics. Antibiotics should be taken for the entire time they are prescribed, even though the symptoms may disappear.
6. Increase your fluid intake enough that you notice an increase in urination.
7. Apply moist heat to the breast for 15 to 20 minutes before nursing or pumping and intermittently between feedings.
8. Monitor your temperature. A mild pain reliever such as acetaminophen (Tylenol) or ibuprofen (Motrin, Advil) may help reduce your fever and discomfort.
9. Consider taking vitamin C. Some women report that a dosage of 1,000 milligrams four times a day speeds healing and recovery.
10. After you have completed a course of antibiotics, watch for symptoms of yeast growth in the baby's mouth and diaper rash caused by yeast (see "Thrush Nipples," page 108).

Breast Abscess

On very rare occasions, a breast infection develops into an abscess. A breast abscess is an accumulation of pus walled off within the breast. It may occur when a mother stops nursing during a breast infection, when treatment for mastitis is delayed, or when a mother has trouble fighting a breast infection because she is anemic.

A breast abscess should be suspected whenever mastitis symptoms last for more than a couple of days and a lump persists. The lump may be hard or soft but does not change with nursing. An abscess must usually be drained by a physician, either in an office or a hospital. After it is drained, recovery is rapid.

Some doctors are willing to avoid surgical drainage by performing a series of needle aspirations, by which a needle is inserted into the abscess and the pus is withdrawn into a syringe. This is much less invasive than opening the abscess to drain over a period of a couple of weeks.

The development and treatment of an abscess can be traumatic. You may be advised to stop nursing entirely, or you may doubt yourself whether you should continue. Although you need not abandon nursing completely, you may be advised against nursing from the affected breast for the first few days after it is drained. In the meantime, you can rent a clinical-grade electric pump to maintain your milk flow until the baby resumes nursing on both sides. The incision may leak milk for a short while, but it will heal and close over. I developed an abscess six weeks after giving birth and went on to nurse successfully without any further difficulties.

Breast Lumps

Lumps in the breast are very common during the early weeks and are usually related to lactation.

The breast may feel generally lumpy when it is overly full or engorged. A tender lump that arises suddenly is usually a sign of a plugged milk duct or, when it is accompanied by fever and flu-like symptoms, a breast infection. A lump that appears just before nursing and seems to get smaller or disappear afterward is probably a small cyst that fills with milk.

Whenever a lump shows no change in size for longer than a week, it should be examined by a doctor. It is probably a harmless cyst or benign tumor; cancer is rarely the cause. But some breastfeeding women with persistent lumps have been found to have breast cancer, so see your doctor for a thorough breast exam as soon as possible. If further diagnosis is recommended, you don't need to wean your baby, although a doctor unfamiliar with the lactating breast may recommend doing so.

Some mothers may need a mammogram, ultrasound, MRI, or breast biopsy to rule out breast cancer. Mammograms and ultrasounds can be performed while you are nursing, but they are best done on an empty breast, so drain the breast as completely as possible just prior to these procedures. When a mother needs a breast MRI, the contrast agent used is generally considered safe to allow her to resume nursing after the procedure. Needle biopsies, both fine-needle and core biopsies, can also be done while a mother is nursing, but mothers are often told to wean because a biopsy can cause a milk fistula. In reality, fistulas are very rare. Any necessary incisions should be done so as to avoid the nipple and areola, especially the lower outer border, to keep from injuring the fourth intercostal nerve. A radial (horizontal) incision is also recommended. The use of local anesthesia is safe for immediate nursing or pumping, and bottle or cup feeding the baby afterward is safe. In fact, the breast should be kept well drained after the procedure by nursing or pumping. Pumping may be preferable if there is much blood coming through the milk—blood can be irritating to the baby's stomach, so he might vomit up the milk.

Consider getting a second opinion whenever drastic measures are recommended.

Leaking Milk

See "Survival Guide: The First Week," page 47, for basic information on leaking, dripping, and spraying milk.

After a few weeks of nursing you may notice that leaking diminishes or stops entirely. This should not be a cause for concern so long as the baby is nursing frequently and gaining weight.

If continuing leakage becomes bothersome, you might want to try stopping it by pressing your wrist or the heel of your hand against your nipples whenever they start to drip. You might also try LilyPadz, sticky silicone pads that can be worn with or without a bra. If leaking at night continues to be troublesome, you might try nursing the baby just before you go to sleep.

Overabundant Milk

Some mothers seem to produce too much milk. Besides feeling weary of the jokes about being able to nurse twins, you may feel uncomfortably engorged much of the time. Leaking and spraying may be bothersome. Your baby may gasp and choke as the milk lets down.

Most women find this less of a problem after the first two months of breastfeeding. In the meantime, nursing your baby on just one side at each feeding should make your breasts feel more comfortable. When your baby is draining your breasts more completely, they will feel less engorged, even though each is nursed on less often. Decreasing your fluid intake is not recommended. Nor is wearing plastic breast shells or pumping after or between feedings, either of which would probably increase, not decrease, milk production. If your baby has difficulty nursing because the milk lets down forcefully, see "Pulling Away from the Breast," page 122. Refer to "Overabundant Milk," page 117, if you continue to produce milk in overabundance after two months.

Lopsided Breasts

When one breast receives more stimulation than the other, milk production in that breast increases, commonly resulting in a lopsided appearance.

Providing more stimulation to the smaller breast will usually even out the size difference between the two. Start each feeding on the smaller side for a day or so. If your baby nurses there for only a few minutes, encourage her to take the smaller breast again after she has nursed at the fuller one. As soon as your breasts become closer in size, you can begin alternating the breast at which the baby begins each feeding.

Nausea or Headache

Rarely, a new mother experiences nausea when nursing her newborn. This is thought to be a gastric hormonal response to suckling. Eating something before nursing may help. Fortunately, nausea generally decreases in severity and frequency as nursing is established, and the problem usually disappears completely by six to eight weeks after birth.

Headaches in new mothers have various causes. A woman who has had spinal or epidural anesthesia may suffer from a severe headache whenever she raises her head. This occurs when spinal fluid, which cushions the brain, has escaped from the spinal canal, causing the brain to sag down into the opening at the base of the skull. Remaining in bed, increasing fluid intake, and drinking beverages containing caffeine may help. When spinal headaches continue for more than a day or two, some doctors offer a "blood patch," by which they inject the mother's own blood into the spinal canal. This often produces immediate relief.

Several case reports in medical literature have concerned "lactational headaches." These occur during feedings as the milk lets down and may be related to the hormone oxytocin. Some writers have said that pain relievers such as acetaminophen (Tylenol) and ibuprofen (Motrin, Advil) are helpful and that these headaches gradually become less severe and stop by two months after birth. But other writers have described cases in which relief came only with weaning.

Another type of headache associated with lactation occurs when one or both breasts are overfull. This type of headache may be a sign of an impending breast infection. Relief comes from draining the breasts well and heading off mastitis.

Other causes of headaches include a drop in hormones in the first week postpartum; low blood sugar; eye, dental, or sinus problems; allergies; or migraine.

Regardless of the suspected cause of your headaches, you may want to consult with your doctor or a neurologist if they are frequent or severe. Keeping a headache log can be helpful in determining a diagnosis.

Depression and Anxiety

Many new mothers experience moodiness, mild anxiety, or an occasional "blue" day during the first two weeks after delivery. These feelings are due to the sudden hormonal changes that follow birth, fatigue from labor and lost sleep, and the stress that becoming a mother entails. But when emotional symptoms are severe, when they continue beyond the first two weeks after birth, or when they start later and last for more than two weeks, they may indicate postpartum depression or anxiety. Many new mothers who complain that they are depressed or anxious are told that their feelings are normal and to be expected. This is not true. Postpartum emotional disorders are often misunderstood or unrecognized by family, friends, and health professionals.

As many as one out of every nine or ten new mothers experiences postpartum depression, postpartum anxiety, or both. Much rarer is postpartum psychosis, characterized by delusions, hallucinations, or extreme mental confusion. Postpartum emotional disorders are more common in women who have had a stressful pregnancy or difficult birth, previous psychological problems, or relationship difficulties. Occasionally, a thyroid disorder may mimic postpartum depression.

Symptoms of postpartum depression or anxiety usually include several of the following:

- Change in eating habits (poor appetite or overeating)
- Change in sleep pattern (difficulty falling or staying asleep, oversleeping)
- Tenseness, nervousness
- Panic attacks with physical symptoms such as shakiness, palpitations, shortness of breath, or lightheadedness
- Fatigue or lack of energy
- Poor concentration, forgetfulness, or confusion
- Crying every day
- Feelings of hopelessness

- Withdrawal, lack of interest in usual activities
- Excessive worry or guilt feelings
- Recurrent disturbing thoughts or compulsive behaviors that cause distress or take up a great deal of time
- Failure to keep appointments

Symptoms that call for immediate assistance from a mental-health professional include these:

- Thoughts of suicide
- Fears of harming the baby
- Sounds and voices heard when no one is around
- Thoughts that seem not your own or out of your control
- Sleeplessness lasting 48 hours or longer
- Inability to eat
- Inability to care for the baby

There are many helpful books available on the topic for mothers suffering from postpartum depression or anxiety. I especially like This Isn't What I Expected: Overcoming Postpartum Depression, by Karen Kleiman and Valerie Raskin (see "Suggested Supplemental Reading," page 182). 414). Many women with mild cases have helped themselves without professional assistance. Try the coping measures that follow.

COPING MEASURES FOR DEPRESSION AND ANXIETY

1. Tell your partner, a supportive friend, or a relative how you are feeling. Although some people may not understand, you may find valuable support close by.
2. Talk to your doctor or midwife about how you are feeling. Ask about blood tests to make sure something else, such as a thyroid disorder, isn't the problem.
3. Call Postpartum Support International (800-944-4PPD) to find out whether there is a postpartum support group in your area. Or visit www.postpartum.net and click on "Get Help."
4. Make getting extra rest a priority; being tired makes depression and anxiety worse. Nap when your baby naps. Maximize your baby's sleep stretches at night by feeding him every two to two and a half hours during the day and evening.
5. Enlist the help of others to relieve you of some mothering and household duties. Eliminate or lessen your daily chores until you are feeling better. If you want to do some chores, set minimal goals for yourself.
6. Maintain a well-balanced diet. If you have little appetite, fix small, nutritious snacks for yourself throughout the day. Avoid all caffeine and sugary foods and beverages; these are associated with worsening symptoms. Increase your intake of foods made up of complex carbohydrates, such as whole-grain breads and cereals, potatoes, rice, and pasta. Eat more fruits and vegetables. Using powdered milk or yogurt, wheat germ, and fruit or juice concentrate, you can make nutritious blender drinks.

If you find it difficult to prepare food for yourself throughout the day, your pharmacist can recommend a high-calorie nutritional supplement such as Ensure or Sustacal.

7. Consider increasing your intake of the long-chain omega-3 fatty acids DHA (docosahexaenoic acid) and EPA (eicosapentaenoic acid), which have been shown to help prevent and remedy postpartum depression and other mental problems in new mothers. The main dietary source of DHA and EPA is fish, but you would have to eat a great deal of fish every week to achieve the necessary levels. Kathleen Kendall-Tackett, a psychologist, suggests taking omega-3 supplements, which can be found at almost any drugstore or health-food store. To prevent depression, she recommends 200 to 400 milligrams of DHA daily. To treat depression, she recommends 1,000 to 2,000 milligrams of EPA daily. These levels are recognized as safe by the U.S. Food and Drug Administration.

8. Try to take time with your appearance every day. When you get up, make a point of getting dressed, fixing your hair, and putting on a little makeup, if you like it. Pamper yourself with a facial, a new hairstyle, or something new to wear. Looking good may help you feel better about yourself.

9. Get some exercise every day. Many people find that exercise has an antidepressant effect. Join an exercise or dance class; many offer free childcare. Take a brisk walk every day with or without the baby.

10. Nurture yourself as much as possible. Take long bubble baths, get a massage, ask your partner to hold you, spend the afternoon watching a video or reading a light novel.

11. Make an effort to spend time with other adults. Invite friends over, join a postpartum group, or make friends with other mothers from your childbirth class. Your childbirth instructor may have additional suggestions. If you have just moved to the area, ask at your pediatrician's or family practitioner's office about social resources for new parents.

If your distress is severe or unrelieved by getting rest and other instituting copingthese measures, consider seeking professional help. Low-cost mental-health care is available in most communities. If cost isn't an issue, ask your doctor, midwife, or childbirth educator to refer you to a therapist, ideally one who has a special interest in postpartum mental illness.

Depending on your symptoms, a therapist may recommend medication. Some antidepressants are safe to use during nursing; others may not be. Safe antidepressants include sertraline, which is sold under the trade name Zoloft; nortriptyline (Pamelor); and paroxetine (Paxil). All of these are also available generically. When nursing mothers take one of these drugs, it is usually undetectable in their babies' blood.

You may be tempted to try St. John's wort, a popular herbal remedy for depression. This herb, however, has not yet been proven safe to use during breastfeeding.

Unfortunately, many doctors who recommend that women wean their babies before taking antidepressants do so because they don't know about recent studies on the safety of particular drugs during breastfeeding. See the LactMed database at www.toxnet.nlm. nih.gov for more information. You may need to share this information with your doctor before coming to an agreement about what is best for you and your baby.

Dysphoric Milk Ejection Reflex (Bad Feelings While Nursing)

Some nursing mothers experience negative emotions beginning just before their milk lets down and continuing from several seconds to as long as a minute or two. This newly recognized syndrome, called dysphoric milk ejection reflex (D-MER), is apparently caused by a sudden drop in dopamine, a hormone and neurotransmitter.

Mothers with D-MER variously describe a sinking feeling in the stomach; a low mood; a brief feeling of hopelessness, depression, apprehension, or dread; "an urge to get away"; or simply "a yucky feeling." A few mothers experience feelings of impatience, frustration, agitation, or anger. The feelings quickly disappear after the milk releases but may recur as the milk lets down throughout the feeding.

D-MER is not postpartum depression or a psychological response to breastfeeding; it is a physiologic response. Happily, many things can help with this problem. Some women just distract themselves while nursing. Others get relief by keeping well hydrated, exercising, sleeping more, or taking small amounts of beverages with caffeine. Nutritional supplements such as omega-3 fatty acids and evening primrose oil may also relieve symptoms. The prescription antidepressant bupropion (the active ingredient in Wellbutrin) may be helpful as well. The website at www.d-mer.org is full of helpful information on managing D-MER.

CONCERNS ABOUT THE BABY

Spitting Up and Vomiting

Spitting up small amounts of breast milk is common; some babies do this after almost every nursing. Recently, it has become common for doctors to diagnose these babies with gastroesophageal reflux, or GER (see "Fussiness, Colic, and Reflux," page 123).

Occasionally a baby may vomit what seems like an entire feeding. Although there may be no apparent cause, this can sometimes be traced to something the mother recently ate. Vomiting can also be a sign of infection. You will want to notify your doctor if the baby has a fever or if the vomiting continues.

When a baby continues vomiting forcefully after most feedings, you should suspect that either he is sensitive to something in your diet or he has pyloric stenosis, a muscular obstruction of the bottom part of the stomach that typically develops at about two to four weeks of age. It is thought to occur in 4 of every 1,000 babies. Although this condition is most common in first-born males, it can occur in females, and one study found it is more common in babies with an allergy to cow's milk. Typically the vomiting becomes progressively worse; the baby eventually stops gaining weight, or loses weight, and may become dehydrated. In the breastfed infant the condition may go undiagnosed longer than in the bottle-fed infant, since breast milk is digested much more easily than formula. The baby's weight may not be affected until the obstruction becomes nearly complete. Frequently, waves can be seen moving across the baby's lower abdomen from the left side to the right just after a feeding and prior to vomiting. X-rays confirm the diagnosis.

The obstruction is corrected with a relatively simple surgical procedure. Breastfeeding can resume within a few hours after the obstruction is removed. At this time breast milk is especially good for the baby because of its digestibility. Some mothers notice a temporary reduction in the milk supply after the baby's surgery. Rest, frequent nursing, and switching the baby from side to side during the feeding usually reverse this situation.

Pulling Away from the Breast

Babies pull off the breast while nursing for a variety of reasons. Often it is because they have had enough to eat or they need to be burped. If your baby has a cold, she may pull away because she is having trouble breathing through her nose. Try to position her so her head is more elevated during nursing. A warm-mist humidifier can be helpful in thinning nasal secretions, as can saline nose drops. You can also use the NoseFrida (see page 106) to remove excess nasal discharge from the baby's nostrils.

Some babies pull away from the breast gasping and choking as the milk suddenly lets down. This is usually a temporary problem; the baby gradually learns to keep up with the rapid flow of milk. In the meantime, positioning the baby differently may help. Try sitting the baby up, using the football hold, or lying on your back with the baby's head over you. You can also try laying the flat of your hand against the breast and pressing inward until the flow of milk seems to subside. Some mothers manually express or pump milk until the initial spray has subsided, but this could work against you by increasing the overall production of milk, which would strengthen the let-down response.

If your baby pulls away from the breast and cries or refuses to nurse, see "Refusal to Nurse," which follows.

Refusal to Nurse

If your baby pulls away from the breast crying or refuses to nurse, don't assume he is ready to wean. There are a number of possible reasons for such behavior, but when it persists, it can frequently be traced to certain foods in the mother's diet to which the baby is sensitive. Typically this behavior starts when the baby is about two weeks old. He may also act fussy and have very frequent, sometimes greenish stools. Other symptoms may include gassiness, redness around the rectum, a mild rash anywhere on the body, or a stuffy nose. Fussiness while nursing and refusal to nurse may occur sporadically or may increase as the day goes on. Although the baby refuses the breast, he may eagerly take breast milk from a bottle. The reasons for this are unclear.

Babies with gastroesophageal reflux also sometimes refuse to nurse. When accompanied by frequent spitting up and fussiness, refusal to nurse is most likely caused by a painful irritation of the esophagus.

A baby who has developed a yeast infection, or thrush, may also become fussy at the breast and refuse to nurse. Besides having a characteristic white coating on the insides of his lips, cheeks, or both, the baby with thrush may be gassy. There may also be a bright red, dotted or peeling rash around the baby's genitals or on your nipples. Your nipples may burn or itch.

Babies with ear infections also sometimes fuss at the breast and refuse to nurse. Although ear infections are less common in breastfed than in formula-fed babies, especially in the first two months after birth, even in this period an ear infection may accompany or follow a runny nose.

Occasionally a baby will refuse to nurse because his mother is wearing perfume or a scented deodorant.

When a baby has been fed supplemental formula and the milk supply has lessened, he may lose interest in the breast, preferring the immediate flow from the bottle. He may fuss and cry when his mother tries to breastfeed him.

TREATMENT MEASURES FOR WHEN THE BABY REFUSES TO NURSE

1. As long as your baby refuses to nurse, express your milk every two to three hours so your supply will not be affected. Use a clinical-grade rental pump or a near-clinical-grade personal pump (see page 140). Feed the baby by bottle.
2. See the next section, "Fussiness, Colic, and Reflux."
3. Check your baby's mouth and your nipples for signs of thrush. See "Thrush Nipples," page 108.
4. If you can find no reason for your baby's irritability and refusal to nurse, have a doctor examine the baby.

Fussiness, Colic, and Reflux

You may be surprised to learn how much crying a baby can do and how uncomfortable it can make you feel. The sound of a baby's cry is intended to be distressing so adults will be alerted to his needs and answer them.

Many mothers tend to blame themselves for their babies' crying, wondering if their inexperience, nervous feelings, or milk supply is somehow responsible. Keep in mind that most babies fuss and seek out the comfort of the breast when they are tired, bored, lonely, or uncomfortable as well as when they are hungry, and that all babies have fussy periods during appetite spurts.

If you are worried that the baby is not getting enough milk, have him weighed. A weight gain of an ounce a day or more means your baby is getting enough milk (see "Underfeeding," page 73).

Some babies are extremely irritable during the early weeks, with periods of intense crying. If your baby's crying makes you feel that something is wrong, trust your instincts. By all means have your baby examined by your doctor.

Outlined below are common reasons that babies cry and suggestions for relieving their distress.

Missing the womb. Harvey Karp, a California pediatrician, theorizes that much of the fussing babies do in the early weeks results from missing the uterine environment. In The Happiest Baby on the Block: The New Way to Calm Crying and Help Your Baby Sleep Longer, Dr. Karp suggests that parents calm their babies through the five Ss:

Swaddling. Many societies have used this technique to imitate the secure feeling of the womb during late pregnancy. A baby is wrapped tightly in a thin blanket with his arms at his sides. Securing the arms and hands keeps the baby from flailing them and makes him more receptive to the other four calming techniques.

To swaddle your baby, lay the blanket out flat, turn in a corner, and place the baby's neck on the folded edge. With the baby's right arm straightened at his side, pull the right corner of the blanket tightly over his body, and tuck it under his lower back on the left side. With his left arm straight at his side, pull the bottom corner of the blanket up over the right arm and shoulder and tuck the blanket under his right side; don't worry about scrunching the baby's legs. Now wrap the left side of the blanket snugly across his body.

Side or stomach position. Although it is now known that laying a baby to sleep on his stomach raises his risk of succumbing to sudden infant death syndrome (SIDS), laying a baby on his back tends to make him startle—to extend his arms and cry out as if he feels he is falling backward. To prevent startling—or the Moro reflex, as it is sometimes called—swaddle the baby and lay him down to sleep on his side, or let him rest on his stomach over your lap or shoulder.

Shushing. Loud white noise calms a baby because it sounds like the flow of blood from the placenta. The louder a baby cries, the louder the shushing he needs. Hair dryers and vacuum cleaners work as well as vocal shushing sounds.

Swinging. Swinging is also reminiscent of uterine life. The swinging should be in rapid, small movements back and forth with the baby face down across your lap. You can swing your baby by wearing him as you walk, by rocking him, or by using a baby swing after the baby is one month of age (see "Coping Measures for Fussiness, Colic, and Reflux," page 123).

Sucking. You can calm a baby who is upset but not hungry by either nursing or offering a pacifier. If your baby seems to need a great deal of comfort sucking, a pacifier may be appropriate. You can introduce one when your baby is between two and six weeks old. Before two weeks a pacifier could interfere with the establishment of breastfeeding, and after six weeks your baby might be much less willing to accept it.

Appetite spurts. You will probably notice that your baby is more fussy at around two to three weeks and again at around six weeks, when most babies experience appetite spurts. During an appetite spurt a baby nurses more frequently for a few days, and this stimulates an increase in milk production. Fussiness in the late afternoon or evening is typical.

The baby's temperament. Every baby is born with her own distinct personality. Some babies tend to be quiet, whereas others are more active. Some babies are highly sensitive to their surroundings and overreact to any sudden stimulation. They are tense, jumpy, and often fussy. They may go almost instantly from sleepy or calm to full-blown crying. Once crying, they may be difficult to soothe. Although some of these babies need to be carried around or entertained continually, others may actually resist being held or cuddled.

Learning how to mother a highly sensitive baby takes time and patience. You will soon develop a sense of what your baby enjoys and what she does not, how much stimulation she can tolerate and how to help her settle down. If your baby does not enjoy touching, try not to take it personally. With time and a gradual increase in physical closeness, she will eventually be able to tolerate and enjoy being held. Most babies outgrow their early fussy months and grow to be happy children.

Diaper rash. A baby may fuss a lot if she has a diaper rash. At each diaper change for an entire day, gently wash the baby's bottom and apply a zinc oxide ointment (such as Desitin). Expose the baby's bottom to the air as much as possible and leave off disposable diapers or plastic pants. The rash should improve dramatically, unless it is caused by yeast (see the following section).

If the baby's stools are green, he may be reacting to certain foods in his mother's diet. See "Colic and Reflux," below.

Yeast infection. Although common in infants, yeast infections are frequently overlooked as the cause of excessive fussiness. A baby with a yeast infection usually shows signs in his mouth—on his inner lips or cheeks, and sometimes also on the tongue. This is known as thrush. The baby is typically very gassy, as the yeast is frequently present in the intestinal tract as well. The yeast may also cause a dotty, red rash or a peeling rash that resembles a mild burn, typically in the genital area. The mother's nipples are often reddened; they may show a rash, and they may itch or burn. One nipple may be more affected than the other.

Nystatin suspension (Mycostatin) is usually the drug of choice when a baby has a yeast infection. Because the nystatin is swallowed, the yeast in the bowel is usually eliminated. Sometimes, however, a diaper rash appears only after treatment with the oral medication, and in other cases a rash gets worse during the first few days of treatment. Nystatin ointment can be used to treat both the mother's nipples and the baby's diaper rash.

The other common oral medication, gentian violet, kills only yeast in the mouth and therefore is not recommended for the baby who is fussy and gassy, unless nystatin seems ineffective after several days of treatment.

See "Thrush Nipples," page 108, for a complete discussion of treatment measures for yeast infections.

Colic and reflux. Colic is a catchall term for unidentified infant discomfort characterized by periods of intense crying and apparent abdominal pain. Although the causes of colic have been much debated over the years, doctors have often dismissed it as something parents must simply endure until the baby is three to four months old, when the symptoms are expected to lessen or disappear. In the meantime, the baby is unhappy, and her mother may wonder if breastfeeding is to blame.

Recently, many babies who might in the past have been labeled colicky have been diagnosed instead with gastroesophageal reflux, which is also called GER or simply reflux.

Reflux is the backward movement of food and acid from the stomach into the esophagus and sometimes into the mouth and out onto your shirt. Nearly all babies have episodes of reflux; most parents consider it normal for their babies to "burp up" after feedings. Some babies who regurgitate frequently show no apparent discomfort. Others, however, seem to suffer painful heartburn, even if they don't spit up their milk.

The main reason babies spit up is that the lower esophageal sphincter isn't fully developed in infants. Also, babies take in a lot of milk relative to the size of their stomachs, and many also swallow a lot of air when they nurse or suck on a pacifier. When the baby burps, milk may come up with the air.

Breastfed babies generally have fewer and less severe episodes of reflux than bottle-fed babies. Sucking at the breast triggers peristaltic waves along the gastrointestinal tract; these muscular contractions help move the milk down into the stomach and on to the small intestine. Also, human milk digests more completely and almost twice as fast as formula. The less time the milk spends in the stomach, the less opportunity there is for it to acidify before backing up into the esophagus. In addition, breastfed babies are generally fed in a more upright position than bottle-fed babies. Gravity may help to keep the milk and gastric acid in the stomach, where they belong.

Still, breastfed babies can suffer painful reflux. Symptoms of this problem can include sudden or inconsolable crying, arching of the back during feedings, refusing the breast or bottle, frequent burping or hiccuping, bad breath, gagging or choking, frequent throat inflammation, poor sleep patterns, slow weight gain, frequent ear infections, and, less commonly, respiratory problems—wheezing, labored breathing, asthma, bronchitis, pneumonia, and apnea.

Some babies with reflux want to nurse all the time and therefore may grow very fast, although it may seem as if they spit up all the milk they take in. On the way down breast milk is very soothing, as is sucking itself. But if a baby overfills her stomach, her reflux symptoms can worsen. For such a baby, it may be helpful to nurse on one breast at a time; the slower flow of milk may soothe the baby's heartburn without overfilling her stomach. Some mothers have reported that pacifiers help such babies.

Other babies with reflux seem to find nursing painful. They not only cry after and in between feedings, but they fuss at the breast and sometimes refuse nursings altogether. Oddly enough, they may take the same milk from a bottle that they wouldn't take from the breast.

Many parents try to minimize reflux by keeping their babies upright or semi-upright for 30 to 45 minutes after feedings. Recent research has found, however, that putting a baby in an infant seat (elevated to 60 degrees) actually increases reflux. Reflux is reduced, the studies have found, when the baby is laid on her left side or on her stomach. But putting babies to sleep on their stomachs has been associated with a higher rate of sudden infant death syndrome (SIDS). Perhaps the best idea is to carry the baby on her left side in a sling, both to minimize reflux and to soothe the baby with the motion of your body. You might also try laying the baby stomach-down on your forearm; parents say that the pressure on the belly seems to be soothing.

Jostling or other rough or fast movement of a baby after feeding may add to the problem of reflux. Burp the baby before switching breasts, but don't jiggle her. Just hold her over your shoulder or sit her upright, and pat her back gently. Let her suck at the breast until she falls asleep.

Some babies seem to suffer more with lower belly discomfort than with regurgitation and heartburn. Besides crying, these babies' symptoms may include gassiness; stools that are very frequent or green, mucous, or even bloody; and redness around the rectum. A baby may have a stuffy nose or a rash on her face or upper body. She may want to nurse all the time.

> Although streaks of blood in a baby's stool or diaper rarely indicate an emergency, for a parent they are alarming, and when they appear, it's a good idea to call the baby's doctor. In most cases, however, blood in the stool results from either an anal fissure or a food intolerance. An anal fissure—that is, a small tear in the anus—usually results from constipation and straining during a bowel movement. Since exclusively breastfed babies cannot be constipated, anal fissures are unusual for them. A sensitivity or allergy to something in your diet is the more likely cause. Some doctors may say that a baby with bloody stools should be temporarily weaned from the breast and fed hypoallergenic formula instead of breast milk, but this is usually unnecessary. In most cases, the bleeding stops after the mother removes the offending food from her diet and the baby's gut has time to heal.

Something in your diet. Whether or not your baby has bloody stools, if she exhibits colic or severe reflux symptoms every day or nearly every day, you should try writing down everything you have eaten and drunk during the past three days. Include any nutritional supplements or medications. Make notes, too, of any particularly fussy periods the baby has had during the past three days. If you are producing a lot of milk, also have your baby weighed to see how fast she is gaining. A baby who is gaining much more than an ounce a day may be having symptoms of what I call hyperlactation syndrome, which is described on page 130.

Most foods that bother breastfeeding babies, as either intestinal irritants or allergens, fall into one of several major food categories. When a baby has been fussy at particular times, a suspect food can often be identified by looking back one to two meal periods or about two to six hours back. If eating chocolate, say, seems to cause your baby's symptoms, you can try giving up chocolate and see if she does better. But because more than one food may be making your baby fussy, you might be wise to avoid all of the commonly offending foods for a while, and then reintroduce them to your diet one by one. This way, you'll know exactly what bothers your baby.

Completely eliminating all of the following foods for three days may bring speedy relief to your fussy baby. Be sure to check the ingredients in any commercially processed food before eating or drinking it.

- **Chocolate and spices.** The major offender in chocolate is theobromide; even in small amounts, this ingredient is a potent irritant in the digestive tract of many infants. In the example given on page 129, the chocolate frozen yogurt was probably responsible for this baby's (and mother's) difficult night. Many spices and other strong flavorings, including cinnamon, chiles, garlic, and curry, can also bother young infants.
- **Citrus.** A frequently overlooked cause of digestive disturbances is citrus fruits and their juices. Oranges, lemons, limes, tangerines, and grapefruits can all bother a baby's intestines. Other strongly acidic fruits, such as pineapples, kiwis, and strawberries, affect many babies similarly. In the chart, the mother had grapefruit juice at breakfast and pineapple juice in the afternoon. Her baby may have been bothered by these.
- **Gas-producing vegetables.** Certain vegetables can also cause temporary digestive problems for young babies. These include onions, broccoli, cauliflower, Brussels sprouts, cabbage, bell peppers, and cucumbers. Prepared mustard can cause a similar reaction. Onions, an ingredient in so many dishes, can cause gastric upset for a baby even when they are cooked, ingested in small amounts, or eaten as onion powder. The stir-fry dish in the chart contained one of these offending foods.
- **Cow's milk.** Some infants are allergic to cow's milk and cow's milk products, including cheese, yogurt, sour cream, cottage cheese, and ice cream. Researchers have estimated that nearly half of all cases of severe reflux and colic are associated with an allergy to cow's milk. If a baby is truly allergic to cow's milk products, cutting back on milk will probably not eliminate the baby's symptoms. You must eliminate from your diet all dairy products, including those in commercially processed foods like creamed soups, certain types of salad dressings, and puddings; cow's milk may be identified as "casein" or "whey" on the label. You should not feed the baby any infant formula made from cow's milk. The baby in the chart may or may not be reacting to dairy products.

8:30 a.m. Grapefruit juice Prenatal vitamin Granola with milk Toast with butter	**10:30 a.m.–12:00 noon** Fussy, spitting up
12:15 p.m. Roast beef and cheese sandwich, with mayonnaise and lettuce Potato chips Milk	
3:00 p.m. Pineapple juice	**2:00 p.m.–5:00 p.m.** Crying
6:45 p.m. Chicken–green pepper stir-fry Spinach and mushroom salad, Italian dressing Rice Milk	
8:15 p.m. Chocolate frozen yogurt	**11:30 p.m.–2:00 a.m.** Very fussy, vomited

Sample chart of a mother's diet and her baby's reactions

If possible, do without certain medications and dietary supplements while you're avoiding these four food categories. Laxatives taken by a nursing mother can disturb her baby's intestinal tract. Aspirin and the chemical phenylpropanolamine, a decongestant, can make a baby fussy; both of these drugs are in many headache and cold remedies. Certain dietary supplements taken by the mother or given directly to the baby, such as vitamin C, brewer's yeast, and fluoride, have been known to cause colic symptoms. Fluoride is very helpful in preventing cavities, but it is best delayed until the baby is six months old and need be given only if your water supply contains less than 0.3 parts per million.

During the three days of eliminating all the commonly offending foods from your diet, write down what you eat and drink along with observations of your baby. If the baby has particularly difficult times, look back one to two meal periods, or about two to six hours before the symptoms began, and try to identify any suspect foods. You may find that you ate something forbidden without realizing it, or perhaps another food seems to be at fault.

Other foods that can cause reactions include tomatoes, eggs, peanuts and peanut butter, corn and corn syrup, wheat (in breads, crackers, cookies, cakes, and noodles), soy (the basis of some infant formulas and an ingredient in many processed foods), apples, and bananas. If you decide to eliminate any one of these foods, you should continue to avoid the original four food categories, too. More than one food group may be affecting your baby.

If your baby is much better after the three days and having very few fussy periods or other symptoms, try adding milk products back into your diet. Have a lot of milk products early in the day and then watch the baby for 24 hours. If the baby reacts, avoid milk products completely for the next couple of days.

After this period, you might experiment with small amounts of milk, cheese, yogurt, or ice cream to see which of these, if any, your baby can tolerate, and in what quantity. Although some babies cannot tolerate any milk products, others do fine when their mothers have hard cheese, and some can tolerate small amounts of any milk products as long as their mothers take them only once every few days. (If you must cut dairy products from your diet completely, be sure you are taking sufficient calcium in another form; see page 94.)

After you have established which dairy products are safe, and in what quantity, add another food category to your diet every few days. Eat a lot of the food in question. If the fussiness recurs, eliminate the offending food category from your diet again. Continue adding food categories until you have tested all the foods that you had eliminated. Again, more than one food may be a problem for a very sensitive baby.

If these measures do not relieve colic, consult your doctor.

Hyperlactation syndrome. Researchers have also identified a kind of colic that is characterized by gassiness, frequent stools, spitting up, and general discomfort and fussiness (Woolridge and Fisher, 1988). Although these babies may seem to be sensitive to something in their mother's diet, they show little or no improvement with the elimination of suspect foods and beverages. Typically these babies nurse frequently from both breasts and are gaining more than an ounce per day. Their mothers often have overabundant milk supplies.

Some lactation professionals refer to these symptoms as overactive let-down syndrome. I don't think that let-down is really the problem. More likely, the underlying cause of the colic is the baby's disproportionate intake of low-fat foremilk, the milk that is available early in the feeding. When a baby consumes large amounts of foremilk and little of the fatty hindmilk, his stomach rapidly empties, dumping excess lactose into the bowel. This results in increased gas and colic symptoms.

Relief is achieved by getting the baby to empty one breast at each feeding so that he receives not only the foremilk but the fatty hindmilk, too. Allow the baby to nurse from the first breast until he spontaneously pulls away satisfied; do not interrupt the feeding at any point to switch the baby to the second breast. If this doesn't help, try limiting the baby to one side for one and a half to two hours before nursing on the other side. Some lactation professionals advise limiting the baby to the same breast for several feedings in a row until the colic subsides, but I feel that this is unnecessary. Keeping the baby at just one side per feeding should solve the problem.

Underfeeding

For any number of reasons, you may wonder if your baby is getting enough to eat. He may seem to be nursing all the time, or he may seem especially fussy. Most young infants want to nurse eight to twelve times in each 24-hour period. Nursing this often is normal and seldom reflects a poor milk supply. You can't tell whether your baby is getting enough breast milk by offering him a supplemental bottle of water or formula after nursing. Most babies will take 1 to 2 ounces if it is offered, even when they have had enough milk from the breasts.

The baby is probably getting enough milk if:

- He is nursing at least eight times in a 24-hour period
- He is nursing for 10 to 45 minutes at each feeding and seems content after feedings
- He has several periods of swallowing during each feeding
- Your breasts feel softer or lighter after the baby has nursed
- Your baby is having bowel movements every day during the first month

If any of these statements isn't true of your baby, have him weighed. Even if all are true, have your baby weighed if you need reassurance. The nurse in your pediatrician's office should be happy to do this for you.

Between the fifth day and the end of the third month after birth, a baby should gain an ounce every day. A weight gain of an ounce a day reflects an adequate milk intake. If your baby was weighed at any time after the fifth day, you can see whether he has gained enough by weighing him again now. If he hasn't been weighed since the fifth day, consider that by 10 to 14 days of age most babies have regained their birth weight. If your baby is two weeks old and weighs less than his birth weight, he probably needs more milk. If your baby is two weeks old and weighs more than his birth weight, he is probably getting plenty of milk, unless the baby is being supplemented. If you have any doubt about how much the baby is gaining, weigh him.

Inadequate weight gain usually occurs when a baby has had trouble latching on or nursing vigorously during the period of initial engorgement in the first week, or when nursing has been infrequent. Underfeeding often occurs among the group of mothers and babies described under "Babies Who May Not Get Enough," page 39. This problem can also occur when a newborn has a faulty suck (see "Sucking Problems," page 69), is tongue-tied, or has a high palate; when a mother has used a nipple shield over her nipple for nursing (see page 58); and, certainly, when a baby is sick. Some laxatives, when taken by the mother, can cause a baby to have excessive bowel movements and to lose weight or gain too slowly even if he is taking enough milk. A baby who gains weight slowly or not at all after gaining well at first may be suffering with painful reflux. Some babies with reflux limit their milk intake because of the discomfort of heartburn (see "Fussiness, Colic, and Reflux," page 123).

Usually a baby's failure to latch on or suck well during the early weeks quickly leads to low milk production. The solution is to build the milk supply by pumping after nursing, and to feed the baby the expressed milk along with any necessary formula.

Treatments and tests for colic. Because tests for colic are invasive, many doctors treat the problem without testing for it. They choose from three kinds of pharmaceutical drugs. First are antacids, which neutralize stomach acid without known side effects. Among these, Mylanta and Mylicon are best known for colic and are available over the counter. They contain simethicone, an anti-foaming agent intended to reduce bloating, discomfort, and pain caused by excess gas in the stomach or intestines. The drops are given right after feedings. Rarely do they seem to help.

Second among kinds of drugs for reflux are those that suppress acid production in the stomach. These include cimetidine (Tagamet), famotidine (Pepcid), nizatidine (Axid), ranitidine (Zantac), and the "acid blockers." Medications in the last group prevent any acid production at all. Among these, omeprazole (Prilosec) and lanseprazole (Prevacid) are approved for use in children, although others are some- times prescribed. Since not all infants react in the same way to these drugs, you may have to try several before you find one that works well. It may take about two weeks before you can tell whether a particular drug works.

The third group of medications prescribed for reflux increase motility—that is, they improve the muscle tone of the digestive tract to keep food moving through it. These medications are more helpful in older babies who are eating solid foods; exclusively breastfed babies generally have fast digestion. Bethanechol (Urecholine), erythromycin, and metoclopramide (Reglan) are the motility drugs currently used in the United States. They can cause gastric cramping and diarrhea. Long-term use of metoclopramide in children (that is, over a period of weeks) hasn't been well studied; in fact, there are concerns about its long-term use in adults.

Some mothers turn not to pharmaceutical drugs to ease their babies' colic symptoms but to old-fashioned "gripe water," which has been marketed since the mid-nineteenth century and is today used around the world. There are many brands of gripe water, but they are similarly formulated; most contain different herbs, and some contain sodium bicarbonate. Although some mothers feel that gripe water has helped their fussy babies, a study published in the New England Journal of Medicine found it generally ineffective against colic symptoms.

A new approach to treating colicky babies uses "good" bacteria, or probiotics. In a study published in Pediatrics (Savino et al., 2007), exclusively breastfed infants with colic symptoms who were treated with Lactobacillus reuteri improved within seven days of the start of treatment. At the end of one month, they had reduced their average crying time by 95 percent. During the same period, colicky breastfed babies treated with simethicone reduced their crying time by only 7 percent. By changing the balance of bacteria in the intestinal tract, researchers speculate, probiotic supplementation may reduce the effects of both gastrointestinal infection and allergic disease. Other studies suggest that L. reuteri inhibits pain by reducing the sensitivity of nerves in the intestinal tract.

The probiotics used in the 2007 study were produced by BioGaia, a Swedish company. These drops have been purchased by Gerber and are now called Gerber Soothe Colic Drops.

Medical tests for reflux and other digestive disorders are rarely advised unless the baby shows signs of poor growth, severe choking, or lung disease. In such a case, the best test for severe reflux is the pH probe, in which a tube is put down the baby's throat to measure the acid level at the bottom of the esophagus. Less invasive is the barium swallow, in which the baby drinks a barium mixture, an X-ray is taken, and then the X-ray is examined for any blockage or narrowing of the stomach valves that may be causing or aggravating the condition. The X-ray, however, will not identify whether a baby's stomach contents are more acidic than normal or if the esophagus has been damaged by reflux. Damage to the esophagus is determined through a more invasive procedure, endoscopy with biopsy. All of these tests should be used cautiously; they do not always provide conclusive results, and they are stressful for both the baby and her parents.

When nothing works. Whether your baby has painful reflux or other colic symptoms, the extreme stress of caring for her may make you consider another feeding method in hopes that the symptoms will lessen. Keep in mind that these conditions usually improve without any such change. Switching to formula, in fact, might well make the problem worse instead of better. Continuing to breastfeed will provide important health benefits for both you and your baby and, most important, a strong bond that can help you both get through this difficult time.

Needless to say, a baby with colic or severe reflux may sleep poorly and fuss a great deal. Your baby may need to be held upright most of the time. She may deprive you of sleep and, by refusing the breast, make you feel rejected. The risks of postpartum depression and even child abuse are higher when a baby has severe reflux or colic. Since this can be a very challenging period even for the most stable family, it is important that you get emotional support, find practical help, and limit your commitments until the problem passes.

COPING MEASURES FOR FUSSINESS, COLIC, AND REFLUX

1. Offer your breast—it is a source of comfort as well as nourishment for your baby.
2. Try a pacifier. Pacifiers are soothing to many babies who need a lot of extra sucking, who are fussy, or who have difficulty calming themselves. If your baby won't take a pacifier at first, try different kinds.
3. Be sure to burp your baby frequently while he nurses or sucks on a pacifier.
4. Try swaddling your baby tightly in a light blanket.
5. Soothe both yourself and the baby with a warm bath.
6. Most babies love motion. Try walking or using a baby pack, sling, or stroller. Rocking can also be comforting—borrow a rocking chair if you don't already have one. Most babies are lulled to sleep by car rides.
7. White noise may calm a crying baby. Try helping him sleep by turning on a radio or a recording of a humming car or vacuum cleaner, or by placing an aquarium near the baby's bed. Or put on a white-noise CD. White noise should be quiet, as recent studies have revealed hearing loss in infants exposed to loud white noise.
8. Consider sleeping with the baby, if you aren't doing so already.

9. Consider purchasing infant probiotics, specifically Gerber's Soothe Colic Drops, and give five drops once a day.

10. Take a short break from the baby each day. Your partner might play with him while you take a bath, go for a walk, or visit a friend.

11. Find another mother who has a fussy baby. There's nothing like a friend who really understands. You might also visit www.colicsupport.com, a website for parents with colicky babies.

Another option, particularly if the baby has become frustrated at the breast, is to first bottle-feed and then nurse. "Comfort nursing"—nursing after or between bottle-feedings, or during the night—may be a pleasant experience for both mother and baby.

Detailed information about formula and bottle-feeding can be found in *The Nursing Mother's Guide to Weaning* (see "Suggested Supplemental Reading," page 182).

CHAPTER 5

Expressing, Storing, and Feeding Breast Milk

- Expression Methods
- Expressing Milk for Occasional Separations
- Expressing Milk Before Returning to Work
- Expressing Milk at Work
- Insurance Pumping
- Expressing Milk for a Baby Who Cannot Nurse
- Pumping Exclusively
- Increasing Your Milk Supply While Pumping
- Collecting and Storing Your Breast Milk
- Feeding Your Expressed Milk

THERE ARE A VARIETY OF SITUATIONS in which mothers express milk for their babies. Some mothers, because of complications, need to express their milk full-time during the early days or weeks after birth; those who are struggling with latch-on difficulties or sore nipples, or whose babies are too premature or sick to breastfeed, may find themselves in this situation. Other mothers breastfeed full-time but need to do "insurance pumping" after nursings to maintain or increase milk production and to provide supplemental milk to their infants. Some mothers, for reasons of their own, exclusively express milk and bottle-feed it to their babies by choice. Some mothers express milk only for occasional separations. And, of course, many mothers who return to the workplace express their milk, not only to feed their babies when they are apart but also to maintain their production.

EXPRESSION METHODS

Hand Expression

Although few mothers today consider regularly expressing their milk by hand, manual expression is a technique that every nursing mother should learn. If you need to express colostrum for a newborn, before mature milk production begins, you may well obtain more by using your hands than by using a pump, partly because the tiny amounts of colostrum produced in the hours following birth can get lost in the plastic parts of a pump. After milk production begins, hand expression can soften your breasts so the baby can latch on more easily. If you begin using a pump regularly, doing some hand expression after each pumping can be a good way to ensure complete drainage of the breast and maximize your milk production. And if pump parts get misplaced, batteries die, electricity goes out, your pump breaks, or you find yourself missing a feeding unexpectedly, hand expression may become a necessity.

When a mother is initiating lactation without a nursing baby, pumping and hand expression combined bring in higher volumes of milk than relying solely on a pump. Dr. Jane Morton of Stanford University has created a short video that shows how to use hand expression to collect more colostrum for a newborn who can't yet breastfeed. You can find this video at http://newborns.stanford.edu/Breastfeeding/HandExpression.html. With several practice sessions, most mothers can master manual expression. You might practice on the free side while nursing, after the baby stimulates the milk to let down. Place a towel in front of you to catch the spray as you get started. Or practice while standing in the shower.

To start, position the pads of your thumb and index finger 1 to 1½ inches behind the nipple directly across from each other. Gently press your fingers straight back toward your chest and then together. Relax your fingers, and then repeat these motions several times. Avoid sliding your fingers away from their original position. Once you have the motion down, rotate your fingers around the nipple to empty other areas of the breast.

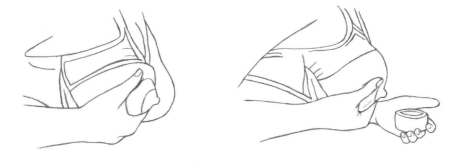

When using hand expression, catch the milk in a cup or any other clean container.

If you begin expressing milk when you're away from the baby, you will probably find that a few minutes of gentle breast massage will help the milk to let down. You can catch the milk in any clean container, but you might prefer a contoured cup specifically designed for the purpose. To get more milk, switch back and forth from one side to the other as soon as you notice the flow lessening. You may be able to save time by expressing milk from both breasts at once, into containers on a table in front of you. Once you have learned the technique, the whole process should take about 20 minutes.

Some mothers actually come to prefer hand expression to pumping. They feel that expressing milk by hand is quieter, more natural, and more convenient than using a pump.

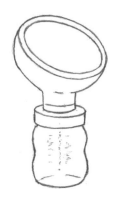

The Hygeia milk expression cup

Pumping

Mothers today are purchasing pumps in record numbers. This is mainly because so many women are returning to work or school within months of giving birth. But even many women who are planning to stay home with their babies see a pump as a necessity, for occasional separations or to allow their partners to participate in feedings.

The great variety of breast pumps available today makes choosing the right pump difficult. I divide pumps into four categories:

- Clinical-grade (rental) pumps
- Personal-use pumps
- Single electric or battery-operated pumps
- Hand-operated pumps

The best pump for you depends partially on how much time you'll be spending away from your baby. If you'll be separated from the baby only occasionally, hand expression or an inexpensive battery- or manually operated pump may be most economical. If you'll be working away from home, say, one and a half days a week, an inexpensive pump may still suffice. If you'll be working full-time, or near full-time, you could find your supply dropping with an ineffective pump. You may want not only a higher-speed, stronger pump but one that will save you time by allowing you to express milk from both breasts at once.

When a full-time worker buys a pump according to price rather than quality, she often finds that her pump is so inefficient that it's useless. Its cycling—the speed at which the pump pulls and releases—is too slow, its suction pressure is too low, or both. She finds she cannot express very much milk. If she uses the pump regularly or often, her milk production may suffer.

The efficiency of a pump depends on two factors: its cycling speed and its suction pressure. The ideal cycling speed is 48 to 60 times per minute. The suction pressure of breast pumps is measured by the movement of mercury in a hydrostatic gauge. The pressure should reach at least 240 millimeters of mercury.

A mother who buys an inefficient pump may not notice the problem at first. Some mothers let down milk easily with nearly any pump in the early days, weeks, or even months, but often after a time a pump seems to lose efficiency. Usually, the efficiency of the pump hasn't changed, but the mother has come to need higher speed and suction.

Sometimes a mother assumes that if she can't pump much milk, she must not be producing much. She worries that she is underfeeding her baby, and she may work at increasing production, when in fact her baby is taking plenty of milk at the breast.

When a mother figures out, sooner or later, that her pump is inefficient, she often has to purchase a second, higher-grade pump, and so she ends up spending more than she would have if she had bought a good pump in the first place. Keep in mind that a high-quality pump is much cheaper than a couple of months' worth of baby formula.

A high price tag, however, is no guarantee that a pump is high-performing. As you will learn later in this chapter, the quality of pumps varies greatly within a particular price range. If you are sure you want to purchase a pump, start by determining the category of pump you need, and then identify a high-quality model within that category. This chapter will help you do just that. If you need extra help, a lactation professional can guide you to the best pump for your situation.

When's the right time to get a pump? Many women do so during pregnancy, but keep in mind that you won't be using your pump until after the baby is nursing well. (If you need a pump in the early days, because of breastfeeding complications, I strongly recommend renting a clinical-grade pump.) You can begin pumping after the first 7 to 14 days postpartum, as your milk supply will most likely be well established by then. Pumping on a regular basis prior to this may cause an oversupply, which can lead to other problems like plugged milk ducts or colic symptoms if the baby is drinking from both breasts and taking in more of the low-fat foremilk than the fatty hindmilk.

Most mothers naturally have more milk during the night and in the morning, so I think that one of the best times to express extra milk is during the morning hours, right after nursing. Pumping in between nursings can be taking some of your baby's next feeding. When you pump in the morning after feeding the baby at the breast, you will most likely get just an ounce or two. But by doing this every day, or nearly every day, your freezer will fill up quickly.

Most young babies will need about 3 ounces per feeding in your absence. So when you pump, place the milk in the back of the refrigerator; when you get 3 ounces, combine the cold milk and then store it in the freezer. Older babies usually need 3 or 4 ounces per feeding. See page 152 for information on milk storage.

Just before the baby is a month old, you'll want to start giving bottle-feedings, of an ounce or so every few days, so that your baby will continue to accept the bottle.

GETTING A PUMP THROUGH YOUR INSURANCE CARRIER

You may know that the Affordable Care Act (ACA) now mandates that mothers covered by private insurance are entitled to breastfeeding support and breastfeeding supplies, including breast pumps. This was signed into law in 2010, and most insurance plans began implementing this coverage on or after August 2012.

Getting a pump from your insurance company can be a bit complicated, but here is some information that can help you. While every plan is different, know that many insurance carriers are still establishing their coverage policies. Unfortunately, there is a great deal of variation in what sorts of pumps are covered, and how they are covered. Because the law's recommendations aren't very specific, coverage varies from insurance company to insurance company. Most plans require women to obtain the pumps from designated vendors, which may or may not offer the pump that a woman hopes for, and that means a mother usually can't simply buy a pump at retail and submit a receipt for reimbursement. Some plans cover only the purchase of cheap manual pumps that may not be effective enough, especially for mothers returning to the workplace. Also, know that there is no co-pay for your breast pump as long as you deal with an in-network provider. Your insurance company will either list these preferred contracted providers on their website, or you can call them for the list. Going out-of-network will usually result in out-of-pocket expenses and less recourse if you are unsatisfied.

Unfortunately, at this time, about a third of insurance plans are "grandfathered" out of having to comply with the ACA because they were purchased before the legislation went into effect. These plans don't have to follow the ACA rules and regulations or offer the same benefits, rights, and protections as new plans. But if the insurance carrier changes any language in its plan, it must then comply with the ACA.

When speaking with your insurance company, talk to them about what you want and need. Some companies offer a double collection electric pump within two months after giving birth, but may offer only a hand pump after two months post partum and up to a year after delivery. Be sure to ask your provider what your "ordering window" is—that is, when you are eligible to place your order and when the coverage ends. Mothers are eligible for a pump only every three years, but you may be eligible for a new collection kit or other parts.

Most insurance carriers refuse to cover clinical-grade rental pumps, which may be needed soon after birth to help mothers establish adequate milk flow because of a sick or premature baby or a breastfeeding complication, like low milk supply. If your insurance carrier does cover one, a written prescription from your baby's doctor and preauthorization is usually necessary. For mothers who need a hospital-grade pump, some insurance companies will cover a standard rental up to the value of the purchase price. In some of these cases, depending on how long the pump is needed, the insurance carrier could actually purchase the breast pump for the mother. The breast pumps must be purchased through a medical equipment company that the insurance company contracts with.

While you are pregnant, try to educate yourself about the many pumps on the market. Later in this chapter, I have included a thorough review of most of the pumps on the market, indicating which ones are commonly offered by insurance carriers, and which get good, mixed, or poor reviews by both mothers and lactation consultants (including myself). It is not too early to contact your insurance provider to see what pumps their durable medical equipment (DME) companies offer to nursing mothers before your baby comes. In this way, you will know which are higher-quality pumps.

Most insurance providers will require you to get your pump from an in-network DME company that they contract with. One recent review of insurance companies revealed that few of them allow mothers to upgrade to a better pump, even if the mother is willing to pay the difference. Some insurance companies without a contracted DME may be flexible if the pump you want isn't available, letting you choose another pump or, rarely, reimbursing your purchase from a retail store. Again, you need to ask for what you want! Because pump benefits vary from company to company, you will need to contact your insurance provider, using the number on the back of your insurance card. The National Women's Law Center can help you if your plan is denying you benefits, unless they are "grandfathered" out. They can be reached by phone at 866-745-5487 or by email at prevention@nwlc.org.

Unfortunately, coverage for lactation services and breast pumps does not cover all women who receive Medicaid or WIC benefits. Twenty-nine states are complying with the Affordable Care Act to provide services and equipment to nursing mothers, but that means that twenty-one states have opted out. You can see if your state's WIC program complies with the ACA at www.advisory.com/daily-briefing/resources/primers/medicaidmap.

Clinical-grade pumps. These piston-driven pumps, built for rental use, cycle automatically about 48 to 60 times per minute and have certain minimum suction pressures of approximately 240 millimeters of mercury. Clinical-grade pumps closely approximate the sucking action of an infant, and most drain the breasts gently as well as effectively. These pumps are available for rent at stations throughout the country.

Medical professionals and pump companies often refer to these pumps as hospital-grade, but usually all they mean is that a pump meets certain electrical and other standards that ensure a pump is safe for hospital use. Know that the designation *hospital-grade* has nothing to do with how well a pump works. I use the term *clinical-grade* to designate pumps of the highest quality.

Clinical-grade pumps are recommended for the following mothers and babies:

- Babies who fail to begin latching on to the breast and sustaining sucking within 24 hours after birth
- Mothers who have no signs of milk production 72 hours following birth
- Mothers who are pumping exclusively or nearly exclusively
- Premature or sick hospitalized newborns
- Babies with poor muscle tone, neurological problems, or birth defects such as cardiac abnormalities
- Mothers who are experiencing breastfeeding problems, such as severe sore nipples, that necessitate temporarily stopping breastfeeding
- Mothers attempting adoptive nursing or relactation
- Mothers estimating their milk supply
- Babies who are refusing the breast, because of colic or a nursing strike
- Mothers who are doing "insurance pumping" after nursings

Probably the finest breast pumps ever manufactured are the large, heavy, internal-piston pumps. To most lactation professionals, they are the gold standard for breast pumps. Unfortunately, most of these pumps are no longer being manufactured. Lighter-weight pumps, with the piston outside the motor case, are more available for rental in most areas but may not be quite as effective as internal-piston pumps.

Double collection kits, which can be purchased at the time of the rental, allow mothers to express milk from either one or both breasts at the same time. Double pumping can significantly cut the amount of time needed to empty both breasts and may stimulate greater milk production than pumping just one breast at a time.

You may be able to find local pump rental stations by calling the toll-free numbers provided by the pump manufacturers. Rental rates vary tremendously, so shopping around can pay off. Rates for long-term, prepaid rental are usually lowest, but in general the cost of a pump rental is far less than the cost of formula-feeding. If your doctor prescribes the use of a clinical-grade pump, your insurance company may cover the cost of the rental depending on your situation.

The Special Supplemental Nutrition Program for Women, Infants, and Children, or WIC, lends external-piston clinical-grade pumps to some of its participants. A mother who qualifies for the program and who needs a pump because she has breastfeeding complications or a premature or sick baby, or because she is working or attending school, may be eligible for the loan of a portable electric pump.

Some larger pump rental stations offer "grant pumps" to a certain number of mothers who can't afford to rent them. If you do not qualify for WIC services and yet don't have enough money to rent a clinical-grade pump, discussing your situation with local rental stations may be worth your while.

Using a clinical-grade pump is usually very simple. Place the flange carefully over the nipple so that the nipple is centered in the middle of the tunnel opening. (If the nipple is off center, it will rub uncomfortably against one side of the tunnel as you pump.) When pumping in the early weeks, many mothers find that a thin coat of lanolin applied around the base of the nipples decreases the friction between the nipples and the hard plastic of the flange. Adjust the suction until it feels strong but not painful. Most mothers start out pumping with low suction and gradually turn up the suction until it feels strong but comfortable.

Personal-use electric pumps. These pumps generally cycle automatically. The best pumps in this category reach suction strengths of 240 millimeters of mercury and cycling speeds of at least 50 per minute. Many, but not all, personal-use pumps have separate controls for adjusting suction strength and speed, which many mothers prefer. Every personal-use double pump comes with a double milk collection kit. These pumps are recommended for:

- Mothers who have normal milk supplies but are separated from their infants nearly every day
- Mothers with normal milk supplies who are experiencing a breastfeeding complication at home (such as a preemie who is sleepy or has a weak suck), but who are still nursing their babies most of the time

- Mothers who have initiated pumping with a clinical-grade pump, have an abundant milk supply, and pump exclusively

Personal-use pumps are not designed for exclusive pumping, particularly in the early weeks. Women who are depending on a pump alone for milk removal usually get off to a better start with a more effective clinical-grade pump.

Many women borrow or are given personal-use pumps from friends or relatives or buy these pumps secondhand. As of this writing, only a few of the pumps in this category—the Hygeia EnJoye Pump, PJ's Comfort Pump, the Melodi Advanced Pump, and the Nurture III Pump—are certified by the U.S. Food and Drug Administration (FDA) as "multiple-user pumps," which can be safely passed on if the new user buys a new collection kit. For reviews of specific pump models, see *The Nursing Mother's Companion, 7th edition* (Harvard Common Press, 2017). Other models in this category are designated as "single-user" pumps, which means they are not to be shared or resold. These pumps cannot be sterilized, so the risk of contamination from viruses transmitted through milk, such as HIV and cytomegalovirus (CMV), cannot be eliminated, even with the purchase of a new collection kit. Airborne viruses can get into the motors of these pumps and cause contamination for the next user. The used pumps that I check out for mothers often harbor mold.

> If you are using a breast pump at high altitudes—2,000 feet above sea level or higher—know that the pump will not generate as much suction as the manufacturer states. Pumps that normally have low pressures will be very ineffective at high altitudes.

It is important to understand, too, that most personal-use pumps have a limited life, so a used pump may not function as well as it did when it was new. Some manufacturers warn that after a year their pumps may not generate as much speed and vacuum as formerly. If you pump every day with a secondhand pump, you may find your milk supply faltering as the efficiency of the pump declines. And if a borrowed pump wears out after the end of the warranty period, you may feel obligated to purchase a new pump for the woman who lent you hers. So borrowing or purchasing a used pump may not be the bargain that it seems. If you own a pump that you used with a previous baby, you will want to check all of the pieces of the kit to be sure the pump will work well for you. Some lactation consultants offer pump "checkups."

Prices vary greatly within this category, as do warranty periods. Purchasing one of the better-quality pumps in this category may save money in the long run, especially if you are going back to work, you will have other children in the future, or both.

As with a clinical-grade pump, using a personal-use pump is fairly simple. Carefully center your nipples in the flange openings. Adjust the speed to about 50 cycles per minute. Start with minimal suction strength, and slowly increase the suction until it feels strong but comfortable.

Single electric and battery-operated pumps. Other pumps that run on batteries or electricity from a wall socket, or both, come in a huge array of styles and models. These pumps are used to express milk from only one breast at a time, which doubles the time it takes to drain both sides. One of these pumps is semiautomatic; that is, the suction is created and released by the user's finger. Other pumps in this category are fully automatic. Fully automatic pumps may remove milk more effectively than semi-automatic ones, but some of the fully automatic pumps in this category cycle much more slowly than the 50 times per minutes ideal for stimulating let-down and emptying the breast completely. Many have poor suction—less than 240 millimeters of mercury—which may also lessen the amount of milk a mother can collect.

Over time, the let-down reflex stops responding well to slow-cycling, low-suctioning pumps—typically the less expensive ones—and this can lead to poor drainage of the breasts and, ultimately, low milk production. As lactation continues, apparently, the breast requires stimulation and drainage that is more similar to that provided by the nursing baby.

In general, these pumps are best for mothers who pump only on occasion. I recommend them only for mothers who have adequate milk production and need to pump no more than five times a week.

To use one of these pumps, center your nipple in the flange opening. If there is a speed setting, try to reach about 50 cycles per minute. Adjust the suction to a strong but comfortable level.

Hand-operated pumps. The final group of pumps comprises those that are hand operated. These pumps are portable and relatively inexpensive; the best are also comfortable and easy to use. Hand-operated pumps are recommended for mothers with adequate milk supplies who need to pump only occasionally, no more than a few times a week.

As with other types of pumps, you'll need to carefully center your nipple in the flange. You may also have to repeatedly squeeze and release a handle or pull and release a cylinder to create suction and control the cycling speed. Familiarize yourself with the manufacturer's directions, and practice to see which techniques work best for you.

The Nursing Mother's Companion, 7th ed. (see "Suggested Supplemental Reading," page 182) has a detailed review of all breast pump models.

EXPRESSING MILK FOR OCCASIONAL SEPARATIONS

If you anticipate that you and your baby will be separated from time to time, you will want to begin expressing milk, by hand or with a pump, once breastfeeding is well established. For most mothers this means sometime after the first two weeks when your baby is latching well at the breast.

Babies will usually happily accept a bottle if it is introduced before they are a month old. They will usually continue to do so thereafter as long as the bottle is offered every two to three days.

If you are offering a bottle just to keep the baby familiar with the artificial nipple, you will need to feed only an ounce or so of milk at a time. Most mothers find they can pump this much after a morning nursing, when production is a bit higher than at other times.

EXPRESSING MILK BEFORE RETURNING TO WORK

If you are facing a return to work or school and so will be missing feedings, you will want to practice hand expression, select a very good pump, or both. If you will be getting a pump, you will probably want to purchase a personal-use double pump that is designed either for personal use or for multiple users.

Most mothers find comfort in having a backup supply of milk in the freezer when they return to work. This extra milk may come in handy whenever you cannot pump as much in one day as you would like or the baby takes more milk than usual.

If your only freezer is a compartment of your refrigerator, collecting just a couple of ounces daily will quickly fill the space. Depending on how much milk you're saving, you may want to search out available space in someone else's deep freezer, or even buy your own. Breast milk will keep for 3 months in the freezer compartment of a refrigerator (with a separate door) and 6 to 12 months in a deep freezer. See page 152 for more information on storing breast milk.

Offer a little of the milk you express to your baby. Offering a bottle frequently and regularly will keep your baby willing to take it if you return to work before he is able to drink well from a cup. Use the oldest milk in the freezer for these practice sessions so that none of your milk becomes outdated. Whenever you offer thawed breast milk to your baby, express some milk to replace what you've taken from your supply.

You will probably discover that you produce the most milk in the night and in the morning. This means that the morning will be a good time to collect extra milk for your baby. Expressing milk right after one, two, or even three of the first nursings of the day typically yields the most milk—for most mothers, 1 to 2 ounces. This milk will have a very high fat content, which will be a bonus for the baby when you are apart.

Mothers whose babies begin a long sleep stretch early in the evening sometimes express milk right before they retire for the night. If the baby doesn't always sleep for a long stretch, however, pumping between nursings may not be a good idea, as you might be taking half of the baby's next feeding.

EXPRESSING MILK AT WORK

If you will be missing one or more feedings while you are away at work or school, you should plan to express your milk. This will help to prevent engorgement and, more important, to maintain your milk supply. The milk you express can be used later to feed your baby while you are away. If you leave your baby for longer than four to five hours three or more times a week and do not express your milk, particularly if your baby is less than eight to ten months old, your milk supply will probably diminish.

How often you should express milk depends on the age of your baby, how long you are apart, and how often the baby nurses while you are together. Babies under four months should nurse at least eight times in 24 hours; emptying the breast this often is necessary to maintain adequate milk production. If your baby is less than four months old, then, plan on expressing milk every two and a half to three hours while away.

Four- to seven-month-old babies typically nurse at least seven times a day. If your baby is this age, express milk often enough so that, with pumping and nursings, your breasts are emptied seven times in each 24 hours. If your five-month-old nurses frequently during the day and twice at night, you may not need to express milk while you work four hours a day, unless you prefer that your baby receive only breast milk when you are apart.

A baby who is eight months old or older may be nursing often or just a few times a day. The decision to express milk at this point depends not only on how much time you spend away from your baby, but also on whether he is eating a wide variety of solid foods and on how you feel about providing formula instead of breast milk.

HOW DOES YOUR FLANGE FIT?

The early weeks at home provide an opportunity to see how well your pump works for you. One question that may arise is whether the flange—the part that fits over the nipple—is the right size for you. If it doesn't fit well, pumping may be uncomfortable, and you may not be able to express milk effectively.

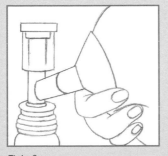

Tight fit

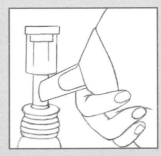

Good fit

Standard flanges are 24 or 25 millimeters wide at the nipple opening. If your nipples are as wide as or wider than a nickel, these standard flanges will probably be too small. Even if your nipples are narrower than a nickel, they may swell in the tunnel of a flange until the fit is clearly too snug. While you're pumping, your nipples shouldn't rub against the side of the tunnel, and the areola, the dark portion around the nipple, should move a bit with each pull. Pumping should be comfortable; experiencing pain on the side of the nipple is another sign that the flange may be too small. Aside from being uncomfortable, an undersized flange may not allow for complete drainage of milk. If you are pumping regularly, incomplete drainage can lead to a drop in overall production. Sometimes when a mother telephones me to ask whether she may need a different flange size, I suggest pumping again 20 minutes after a regular pumping. Collecting more than ½ ounce of milk in the second pumping may indicate that the flange fits poorly. If you are using a Medela or Ameda pump, you can order large or extra-large flanges from the manufacturer. Have a lactation professional check the fit; she may have a larger flange available for sale.

It is important to also understand this: Extended periods of time without complete breast drainage lessen overall milk production. For most women, if the breasts aren't thoroughly drained seven times in a 24-hour period, milk production declines.

This decline in milk supply involves several factors. A lessening in breast stimulation, experts think, leads to lower prolactin levels, the hormone responsible for milk production. Additionally, full breasts that go undrained for long periods of time probably release substances that cause the milk-producing cells to slow or even cease production.

Some people mistakenly theorize that when a woman regularly goes for lengthy periods without nursing or expressing milk, the breasts become "trained" to produce sufficient amounts of milk when she does put the baby to breast. Unfortunately, this is not the case. Neglecting to express milk when apart from the baby leads to an overall lessening of the milk supply. A low milk supply generally leads to a delayed milk let-down, frustration at the breast for the baby, and in many instances premature weaning.

If you decide against expressing milk, your baby will need a commercially prepared formula for missed nursings during the first year.

INSURANCE PUMPING

There are several situations in which it may be important to express milk after nursing a baby. This is called "insurance pumping." Mothers and babies in this category include:

- Babies making the transition to full-time breastfeeding (see page 84)
- Babies born at 37 weeks' gestation or earlier or weighing less than 6 pounds (see page 79)
- Babies who have unusual conformations in their mouths, such as a short frenulum, a high palate, or a cleft lip or palate or both (see page 88)
- Babies who are being fed with the help of a nipple shield (see page 58)
- Mothers who by 72 hours following birth have had no signs of milk production (see page 48)
- Mothers with low milk production (see page 73)
- Mothers whose breasts remain engorged because the baby isn't thoroughly draining them (see page 47)
- Mothers with nipples as large in diameter as a quarter, or larger (see page 71)
- Mothers who have had previous breast surgery involving an incision around the nipple or areola
- Mothers diagnosed with polycystic ovary syndrome (PCOS)
- Mothers with hypoplastic breasts (long, thin, widely spaced breasts that didn't get larger in pregnancy and that may differ markedly from each other in size)
- Mothers in the categories just listed are at risk for low milk production, and their babies are at risk for poor weight gain. In many of these cases, the babies may not be vigorous enough to stimulate and drain the breasts well and to bring in a full milk supply. This is often true with near-term babies and babies making the transition to full-time nursing. A mother may bring in a full milk supply, but if the baby nurses poorly, the supply may plummet. In other situations, the baby may suck well, but the breasts

may need more stimulation and emptying than the baby can provide. Examples are mothers with large nipples and mothers who have had breast surgery. In these cases, pumping right after nursings can be necessary to bring in an abundant supply, as well as to insure that the baby receives plenty of milk.

Generally, double-pumping for 5 to 15 minutes with a clinical-grade pump right after nursing will drain the colostrum or mature milk remaining in the breasts. When a mother pumps after each nursing, not only does her milk supply usually increase, but her baby begins receiving more milk. One pediatrician put it this way: "Insurance pumping makes the breast perform more like a fire hydrant and less like a garden hose."

Newborns in the insurance-pumping categories need to be carefully monitored for signs of adequate milk intake. If your newborn loses 10 percent of her birth weight (see Appendix) or if she fails to gain an ounce a day after five days of age, you'll need to feed her some or all of the milk that you collect by pumping. If you can't collect enough milk, she may also need supplemental formula. In these cases, working with a lactation professional can be very helpful.

When your baby is gaining weight normally without supplemental breast milk, you can slowly wean yourself off the pump. After doing so, continue to monitor the baby's weight for a short while.

EXPRESSING MILK FOR A BABY WHO CANNOT NURSE

Some mothers must bring in a milk supply without a nursing baby. If your baby is unable to nurse because of a latch-on problem, prematurity, or illness, you will want to start pumping as soon as possible, ideally within hours of delivery, so your baby receives plenty of colostrum. Colostrum is especially beneficial because it has such a high concentration of protective antibodies.

The nursing staff should provide you with a suitable pump and instructions for collecting and storing your milk. Most maternity units have a clinical-grade breast pump available; this is the type of pump you want when you must pump around the clock. If your baby is being transferred to another hospital for care, ask the transport team about their procedures for storing and transporting your milk. If you will be following the baby to a special-care nursery in another city, try to get a pump to take along with you.

It is very important that you have the right size flanges for pumping. Some standard pump flanges are too small for many mothers. If your nipples are swelling in the tunnels, and especially if pumping is painful, the flanges may be too small. If they are, your breasts won't drain completely. For advice on choosing the correct flange size, see page 145.

Initially, you may be more comfortable if you apply a thin coat of lanolin around the base of the nipples before starting to pump. If pumping is painful even with lanolin, again, you may need larger flanges.

You may receive differing bits of advice on how often and how long to pump your breasts. Some hospital nurses suggest that women pump every three to four hours during the day and sleep all night. With such limited stimulation, most mothers would find either that they wouldn't bring in an abundant supply or that after a while it would dwindle. Keep in mind that your milk supply depends on the frequent stimulation of your breasts. You should plan on expressing milk as often as your baby would nurse, or at least eight times in 24 hours. Some mothers prefer to express their milk every three hours around the clock, whereas others would rather pump a little more often during the day so they can sleep for longer periods at night. Determine a reasonable schedule for yourself, but do not go more than five hours without pumping.

Studies now suggest that the effectiveness as well as the frequency of colostrum removal in the first three days is highly predictive of how much milk will be produced in the days to follow. Surprisingly, dependence on a pump alone during the first several days may be associated with lower milk production. Dr. Jane Morton and others at Stanford University have found that pumping alone may remove only a fraction of the available colostrum and milk. In this study, mothers who both hand-expressed colostrum and pumped with the Medela Symphony pump collected 80 percent more milk than women who used only the pump. For instructions on hand expression, see page 136. You can see Dr. Morton's technique in the video at http://newborns.stanford.edu/Breastfeeding/HandExpression.html.

If you are hand-expressing for a healthy full-term or near-term baby who is unable to latch on to the breast, you can collect the colostrum in a plastic spoon, which you can then use to feed the baby. If your baby is sick or very premature, ask the hospital staff about using a small container to collect and store colostrum for later use.

Once your milk is in, how much you produce will depend on how much you manage to express. Ideally, you should pump more milk than your baby requires. Building and maintaining a volume of at least 24 ounces per day (or, for twins, 40 to 48 ounces per day) will allow you to have extra milk on reserve should you experience a temporary decline in production—due to stress or illness, for example—during your baby's hospitalization. Having an abundant supply will also help your baby get milk more easily once he is able to latch on to the breast and suck.

You can maximize the amount you collect by massaging or pressing firm areas of the breast while you pump. To see Dr. Morton demonstrate the hands-on pumping technique, go to http://newborns.stanford.edu/Breastfeeding/MaxProduction.html.

It may be easier to massage and compress your breasts if you pump one side at a time. Alternatively, you can wear a hands-free bra, also known as a pumping bustier, which will hold the pump flanges in place (see page 145). A tight sports bra with the centers cut out can also allow you to massage and pump both breasts at once.

After pumping, you can collect even more milk by hand-expressing for a few minutes, alternating breasts several times.

With practice and experimentation, you will develop your own method for collecting the most milk possible. Most mothers find that once they are able to pump 3 to 4 ounces at a time, they can gradually eliminate the other measures to increase milk production.

Whenever possible, provide freshly expressed or refrigerated milk for your premature or sick baby. Freezing breast milk preserves many but not all of its protective substances. You can keep your milk for 24 to 48 hours in the refrigerator (ask the intensive-care nurses for a more precise limit) or for up to three months in the freezer.

Depending on your baby's maturity or general progress, you may find yourself expressing milk for several weeks. It is important that you eat well, get plenty to drink, and rest enough to maintain your own energy as well as your milk supply.

If you notice that your milk production is declining for a few days in a row, you will need to assess the situation and make whatever adjustments are necessary. The most common causes of decreasing milk production are infrequent expression—fewer than eight times in 24 hours— and an inefficient pump. Although a few mothers can maintain a good milk supply while expressing less often than this or while using a non-clinical-grade pump, most can't do so for longer than a few weeks. If you have been using a hand pump or an inexpensive battery-operated or plug-in pump, or even a personal-use pump, rent a clinical-grade pump. Most mothers find that a clinical-grade pump requires less effort to operate and works more efficiently. Using Dr. Morton's methods to increase milk production, as described in this section, may also help improve your overall production.

Occasionally you may notice that your milk production drops when you and your baby have a difficult day. Stress can temporarily decrease a mother's milk supply; this is normal and usually temporary. The following suggestions have proven helpful when this occurs:

- Pump regularly, every two to three hours.
- Take a short nap or a warm bath just before expressing.
- Apply moist heat to your breasts before expressing.
- Massage each breast as you pump, and perform hand expression right after each pumping.
- Ask someone to rub your back between the shoulder blades while you are pumping.
- If possible, hold the baby while you are pumping at the hospital, or keep a photo of your baby with your pump.
- Hold the baby skin-to-skin as much as possible.

PUMPING EXCLUSIVELY

For any of a variety of reasons, a woman may find herself pumping all of her baby's milk and feeding it by bottle instead of nursing. It may be that the baby has been unable to latch on to the breast, or even that the mother prefers to feed her baby this way. Many women have managed to produce enough milk to meet their babies' needs for a year or beyond while pumping exclusively.

Pumping full-time for a baby requires dedication and discipline. Unlike a baby, a pump does not signal for attention, and for most women pumping is more a chore than a pleasure. To feed your baby entirely or mostly on your own milk, however, is to give him an extra-special gift.

If you are exclusively pumping, frequent and effective expression during the first week after birth is critical for establishing an abundant milk supply. Read "Expressing Milk for a Baby Who Cannot Nurse" (page 147), and make sure you have a high-quality, comfortable pump. Starting out with a clinical-grade rental pump is the best way to bring in a full milk supply—about 24 ounces per day during the first month. Since clinical-grade pumps are expensive, women who use them rent them rather than buy them. If your income is low or modest, you may qualify for a rent-free clinical-grade pump through the WIC program. In any case, long-term pump rental is much less costly than buying formula.

A double collection kit, for collecting milk from both breasts at once, makes pumping quicker and is usually more effective in establishing and maintaining milk production. Unless you are given a collection kit in the hospital, you will need to buy one when you rent a clinical-grade pump.

It is essential to pump often—every two to three hours during the day and at least once in the night, or at least eight times in each 24 hours. You must also spend enough time at each pumping to drain both breasts completely, since it is the frequent, thorough drainage of the breasts that signals them to increase milk production and keep it high. Some women can completely drain the breasts by pumping for 10 minutes or less, but others need a longer time. Until you're sure how much time you need, pump until the milk stops flowing and then a couple of minutes longer.

Pumping shouldn't hurt. A properly fitting pump flange allows for the pull and release of the nipple without the nipple's swelling against the side of the tunnel. If the tunnel is too narrow for your nipple, your breast won't drain completely and pumping may be painful. For help in determining whether you need a larger flange, see page 145.

Once you have established a generous milk supply—at least 24 ounces per day—you might invest in your own personal-use pump, such as Hygeia's EnJoye, Medela's Pump in Style, or the Calypso pump. Some mothers, however, are unable to maintain high production with these pumps and continue to require a clinical-grade rental model.

After the first month, most women are able to maintain their production level with seven pumpings in each 24 hours. With less frequent pumping than this, however, most

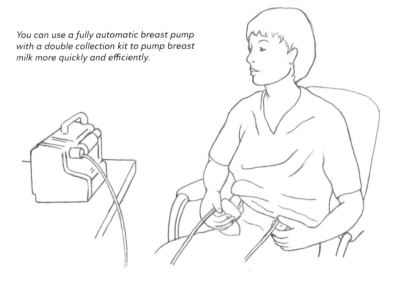

You can use a fully automatic breast pump with a double collection kit to pump breast milk more quickly and efficiently.

women find that their supply drops below the baby's needs. A small proportion of women produce excessive milk while pumping only five or six times in each 24 hours. If you are an overproducer, you can freeze the extra milk for later use.

Mothers who are exclusively pumping especially appreciate products that allow hands-free pumping.

Your milk supply will need to grow as your baby does. From the fifth day after birth until about three months, babies generally gain about 1 ounce per day. After three months of age, their weight gain typically slows to about ½ ounce per day. They require 20 to 24 ounces of milk per day in the first month, and their intake gradually increases thereafter to 28 to 32 ounces per day. Their intake stays at about this level until other foods slowly begin to replace breast milk in the diet.

Bottle-fed babies often drink more than they need for normal growth, even when they're fed breast milk rather than formula. Since overfeeding a baby can lead to obesity later, you may want to keep track of how much milk your baby is taking. These guidelines may be helpful: During the first month, offer about 1 ounce per hour, or 3 ounces every two and a half to three hours. After the first month, offer as much as 1½ ounces per hour, or 4½ ounces every three hours. If your baby seems to want more milk than this, try to keep in mind that babies often fuss when they are overstimulated, tired, or uncomfortable. A breastfeeding mother may put her baby to the breast hourly when he is tired or cranky, but he doesn't get a large meal at each comfort feeding. Carrying your baby or offering a pacifier between feedings may help in calming him. (If your baby is very fussy, see "Fussiness, Colic, and Reflux," page 123.) Learning how to do "paced" bottle-feeding can also help your baby take a more normal volume of milk by bottle. (See page 157 for information.)

If you're pumping out of necessity rather than choice, it may be helpful to know that many babies become able and willing to take the breast despite weeks or even months of bottle-feeding. If your baby has been unable to latch on and suck well, it is still worthwhile to try nursing periodically. A lactation professional may be able to help you.

INCREASING YOUR MILK SUPPLY WHILE PUMPING

Some women who exclusively or frequently pump struggle with low milk production. If your production is lower than the norms specified here, you can take measures to increase it.

1. Be sure that you are not pregnant or using estrogen-containing birth control (combination birth control pills or the vaginal ring with estrogen), which typically lessen milk production. The progestin-only "mini-pill" is usually fine.

2. Consider using a clinical-grade pump and a double-pump kit, if you are not doing so already.

3. Pump or nurse *at least* eight times a day—more if you can manage. Distribute the pumping or nursing sessions more or less evenly during the baby's waking hours. If your baby sleeps a long stretch at night, pump just before you go to bed or very early in the morning. If you work away from home, nurse or pump right before leaving the baby and as soon as you return.

4. If you're not sure whether your pump is draining your breasts completely, try pumping 15 to 20 minutes after a prior pumping. If you get ½ ounce or more at the second pumping, the collection kit, or even the pump itself, may be doing an inadequate job.

5. To be sure your pump is working efficiently, give it a checkup. Check the tubing, connections, rubber diaphragms, and filters. If the diaphragms get small tears, the pump will not work efficiently. If the filters get wet, the suction will stop entirely. A lactation professional may be able to check the pump's suction pressure, which should reach 240 millimeters of mercury. Some pumps are simply not capable of reaching these pressures.

6. Be sure the pump's nipple flanges fit you right (see page 145).

7. Pump at the highest suction possible without discomfort, and at a speed of about 50 times a minute. If your pump doesn't have a speed control labeled with the number of cycles per minute, count the cycles. Pumping too fast or too slowly can reduce the volume of milk expressed.

8. Practice "hands-on pumping," as described on page 148.

9. Consider using Pumpin' Pal Super Shields, which might help you express more milk, especially if your pump has adequate suction.

10. Consider taking herbal products that stimulate milk production, such as fenugreek or blessed thistle capsules, More Milk Plus tincture or capsules, or Go-Lacta (see page 50).

11. If your periods have resumed and you find that your milk production dips when you are mid-cycle until your period begins, consider taking 500 to 1,000 milligrams of calcium and 250 to 500 milligrams of magnesium daily. Take this from the time of ovulation until the day of your heaviest flow.

COLLECTING AND STORING YOUR BREAST MILK

Regardless of whether you have a healthy baby or one who is premature or sick in the hospital, you will always want to take special care when expressing and storing your milk. Wash your hands before handling your breasts or any of the pump equipment. All pump parts that come in contact with the milk or your breasts should be thoroughly washed after each use, with hot soapy water and separately from family eating utensils and food preparation equipment. Use a bottle brush, one with a smaller brush on the opposite end, to reach all the nooks and crannies of the pump parts. (Some mothers buy a second collection kit so they can do the washing at their convenience.) Your daily bath or shower will cleanse your breasts sufficiently.

You can store your milk in plastic or glass feeding bottles or in plastic bags made for milk storage. Plastic bags take up less space in the freezer than bottles do, and you may be able to express your milk directly into the bags. Some mothers use disposable bottle liners, but these can break when the milk freezes and leak when it thaws. Bags designed for storing breast milk are made of thicker plastic, come sterilized, and have a place for writing the date. The main disadvantage of milk storage bags is that they are not reusable. Also, you cannot add fresh milk to a bag of frozen milk or feed the milk to the baby directly from a defrosted bag. The bags are more prone to leakage than bottles, but you can minimize this problem by putting the filled bags into freezer-weight food storage bags.

Some time ago, it was discovered that clear plastic baby bottles made of polycarbonate contain the chemical bisphenol-A (BPA), and that the BPA can leach into milk or other liquid in the bottle. Although most data concerning the safety of BPA come from animal studies, many scientists believe that the chemical can cause behavioral and developmental problems in children. Both the United States and Canada have outlawed the sale of baby bottles containing BPA. Flexible, opaque polypropylene bottles are BPA-free, as are glass bottles. Nearly all bottles and pump parts are now BPA-free.

Unless you are collecting 1- to 2-ounce bottles for practice feedings, store your milk in quantities of 3 to 4 ounces. Place your milk in the back of the refrigerator, at 34 to 40°F, if you plan on using the milk within 72 hours. Freshly refrigerated milk is better for your baby, as it retains more of its live cells than frozen milk. If you wish to add more milk to some that is already bottled, chill the new milk in the refrigerator for about half an hour before adding it.

Many breastfeeding specialists say that milk can be safely refrigerated for up to eight days. Lois Arnold, former executive director of the Human Milk Banking Association of North America and currently the program coordinator for the National Commission on Donor Milk Banking, disagrees. The eight-day rule, she explains, fails to take into account that some mothers' milk may have high levels of bacteria, perhaps because of bacteria on the skin, inadequate cleaning of pump parts, or the use of contaminated water for cleaning equipment. Because you can't be sure that your milk doesn't have high bacterial levels, I recommend keeping it in the refrigerator for no longer than 72 hours. If you will not be using your expressed milk within this time, store it in the freezer compartment of a refrigerator (with a separate door) or in a freestanding freezer. Even milk that has been refrigerated for three days can be safely moved into a freezer.

Lack of refrigeration should not be a problem if you'll be expressing milk when you return to work. One small study found that freshly expressed milk could be kept at room temperature (66 to 72°F.) for up to ten hours without spoiling. However, I recommend keeping your milk chilled in a small cooler with freezer packs if a refrigerator is not available.

Breast milk looks different from dairy milk, especially after storage in the refrigerator or freezer. Your fresh milk may be yellow, white, bluish, or even greenish, depending on what you have eaten and what medicines or vitamins you have taken. Frozen breast milk is usually yellow. Your milk will naturally separate in the refrigerator; the fat will rise to the top. After warming the milk, gently swirl it to mix the layers.

Fresh or thawed breast milk typically has a mild, slightly sweet smell. Occasionally a mother finds that her expressed milk has an unpleasant smell or taste. Certain vitamin or mineral supplements can cause this; so can steroidal nasal sprays. In either case, the affected milk is harmless.

Breast milk can take on a soapy smell if the fat has broken down, freeing fatty acids. Apparently, some women have an excess of lipase, the enzyme that breaks down the fat in milk. Usually they notice the soapy smell after the milk has been refrigerated or frozen, but in some cases the smell develops immediately after expression. Most babies will take such milk without complaint, but the peculiar odor and taste can usually be lessened or eliminated either by chilling the milk before freezing it or by putting it directly into the freezer, and then thawing it in the refrigerator before warming it in a hot-water bath. If these methods fail for you, you can inactivate the enzyme by scalding the milk on the stove—that is, by bringing the milk almost to a boil—and then immediately refrigerating or freezing it. Do not let the milk boil; doing so would destroy its anti-infective properties.

Although freezing destroys the white blood cells found in breast milk, it preserves the many other antimicrobial properties and inhibits the growth of bacteria. Freezing does not affect the nutritional composition of breast milk.

You can safely store your milk in the freezer compartment of a refrigerator for three to six months, provided that the freezer compartment is separate from, not inside, the refrigerator, and that the temperature stays at –4°F. Store the milk toward the back of the freezer, away from the door. If the freezer automatically defrosts, keep the milk away from the walls.

Because the entire amount must be used once breast milk is thawed, you will want to store small amounts, probably 3 to 4 ounces. Regardless of what kind of container you use, leave some room at the top to allow for expansion and to avoid leakage. If you want to add fresh milk to some that is frozen, chill the fresh milk first to keep the top layer of frozen milk from thawing.

Date your containers so that you use the oldest milk first. While bottles are often recommended, you may find that bags made especially for breast milk will take up less space. Using other types of bags is not recommended due to leakage problems. If you will be taking the milk to day care, write the baby's name on the bags as well. Placing the bags in a plastic container will also help keep them safe from breakage.

Better yet, store the milk in a freestanding deep freezer, where the milk will be good for 12 months when the temperature is –4°F. If you don't have a freestanding freezer and you are running out of space in the freezer section of the refrigerator, you might invest in a small one or find a friend or relative who has one that you can store your milk in.

Collecting Milk for a Premature or Sick Baby. If you are expressing milk for a premature or sick baby, you should not only wash the pump parts in hot, soapy water, you should also sterilize them every day. You can boil them in water for 15 minutes or run them through a dishwasher's sanitizing cycle, or you can sterilize them in special bags in a microwave oven: Place all of the parts that come in contact with milk in one of the bags with 4 ounces of water, and microwave for the time recommended on the bag, usually between 1 and 5 minutes.

After collecting your milk, pour it into a sterile container; ask the hospital nursery staff what type they prefer. To avoid wasting milk, ask your baby's nurses how much to put in each container. Freshly refrigerated milk is better for your baby, as it retains more of its live cells than frozen milk, so try to provide fresh milk for your baby whenever possible. Milk for a premature or sick baby can be safely stored in the refrigerator for up to 48 hours (ask the nursing staff for their specific limit).

When transporting your refrigerated or frozen milk to the hospital, pack the containers in ice, or surround them with refreezable ice packs, inside a small cooler. If you're traveling a long distance, keep your milk frozen with dry ice.

Milk for a premature or sick baby should not be frozen or refrigerated after it has been thawed or warmed. Whatever is left over after the feeding must be thrown out.

FEEDING YOUR EXPRESSED MILK

Take your milk out of the refrigerator shortly before your baby is due for a feeding. Gradually, over 5 to 10 minutes, warm the milk to room temperature in a container of warm water. Never warm or defrost milk in a microwave oven or on the stove. Microwaves do not heat evenly, and uneven heating can burn a baby's mouth. Bottles can explode in microwave ovens. In a microwave or on a stove, excess heat can destroy the immunological substances, proteins, and vitamins in breast milk.

When taking milk out of the freezer for feeding, choose the oldest milk; this way you're less likely to end up throwing away outdated milk later. Thaw the milk in any of three ways: Hold the container under warm running water; swirl it in a bowl of warm water; or let it thaw overnight in the refrigerator. Do not thaw milk by letting the bottle sit at room temperature.

When breast milk thaws, the fat separates and rises to the top. Gently shake the bottle to blend the fat back in with the rest of the milk. Use thawed milk within 24 hours. Do not refreeze it.

Mothers often ask whether they can reuse breast milk left over after a feeding. Although there have been no scientific studies on this question, most lactation professionals believe that warmed or defrosted milk can be refrigerated, reheated, and used for the next feeding so long as the baby isn't sick or premature and the milk has not been left out for longer than an hour.

Getting your baby used to a bottle is important if she will be fed by someone else while you are apart. It is best to wait until she is two to four weeks old before introducing a bottle. By this time nursing should be well established, so the bottle should not interfere with the baby's interest in the breast. Many babies refuse the bottle if it is first offered much after they are one month old.

Many kinds of bottles and nipples are on the market, and no one bottle or nipple is best for breastfed babies or more likely to be accepted over another. The best bottles are easy to clean and have accurate measuring indicators. Angled bottles are supposed to make it easier to keep the nipple filled, so the baby doesn't suck in air, but this is just as easy with straight bottles and actually unnecessary (see "Baby-Led or Paced Bottle-Feeding," page 157). Bottles molded into unusual shapes or split down the middle for self-feeding are nearly impossible to keep clean. Some bottles come with disposable liners, which are supposed to cause less air swallowing. They don't.

Most bottles come in two sizes: 4 ounces and 8 ounces. Four-ounce bottles make more sense for babies who are taking only 2 to 4 ounces at a feeding. You can buy 8-ounce bottles later, if your baby begins drinking 4 to 5 ounces at a feeding.

Nipples are made of latex or silicone. Silicone nipples are definitely preferable. Latex has a taste and odor and deteriorates faster than silicone. Latex also tends to break down in the dishwasher and so should be washed by hand. Silicone nipples *can* be washed in the dishwasher.

To introduce a bottle, manually express or pump your milk instead of nursing, and then, if possible, have your partner or someone else feed the milk to the baby. If you do this about three times a week until you go back to work, your baby should continue to accept a bottle. Offering a bottle periodically will also give you the opportunity to practice manual expression or become proficient with your pump.

Parents who stop offering a bottle once the baby has taken it sometimes find themselves struggling with the baby and bottle weeks later. Giving the baby 1 or 2 ounces of breast milk by bottle every few days is very important if you want to avoid problems later.

Should your baby refuse to drink from a bottle, keep trying. The following suggestions may help:

- To avoid wasting your milk, practice with just 1 ounce in the bottle.
- Don't substitute formula for your milk in these practice sessions. Most babies prefer sweet-tasting breast milk to formula.
- Try a variety of bottle nipples. Look for one with a faster flow. Try a tasteless silicone nipple instead of a latex one. Different mothers swear by different brands, including Avent, Playtex, Mimijumi, and Dr. Brown's.
- Try offering the bottle while walking with the baby. Hold the baby facing away from you, and bounce her gently as you walk. This will be easier if you put the baby in a front-facing carrier.
- Try nursing the baby for just a few minutes, and then unlatching her and slipping the bottle into her mouth. If she objects, try again after a few minutes more of nursing.
- Have someone else try; frequently a baby is more confused and upset by a bottle when her mother tries to persuade her.
- As long as the baby is refusing the bottle, offer it a couple of times each day, both when the baby seems hungry and when she is not.
- Do not allow these sessions to become too upsetting for the baby or for you. Trying to force a baby to take a bottle is distressing for everyone and rarely successful. Also, "starving" the baby until she accepts a bottle is somewhat abusive and rarely effective.

Although you want to know before you are apart that your baby will drink from a bottle, the baby who won't take a bottle from Mom may do well when the caregiver offers it. At the age of three months, my daughter, Kate, screamed bloody murder whenever I approached with a bottle, but her caregiver had no problems feeding her when I was away.

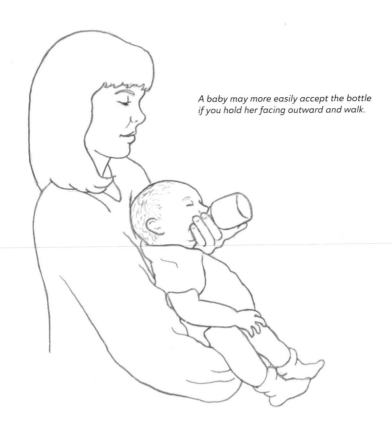

A baby may more easily accept the bottle if you hold her facing outward and walk.

The baby who refuses a bottle may do surprisingly well with an ordinary, unspouted cup, particularly if she is nearing six months or older. A sippy cup may be too much like a bottle for a baby who is continuing to refuse one.

Baby-Led or Paced Bottle-Feeding. When you are feeding your baby your milk by bottle, always hold him in your arms. Let him control the feeding in the ways he does when you nurse him: Wait for him to open his mouth instead of pushing in the nipple. Be patient when he pauses in sucking; don't stimulate him to suck continuously. Even if there is breast milk left in the bottle, let your baby stop drinking when he signals that he has had enough.

A full bottle-feeding should take 7 to 15 minutes. If the feeding takes longer, the nipple flow may be too slow. If the baby chokes frequently, the nipple flow is too fast.

Breastfed babies, in most instances, control the flow of breast milk as they nurse. When you're breastfeeding, the milk may spray as it lets down, and the baby may let go of the breast to prevent himself from choking. After the first let-down, the baby then controls the flow of milk by sucking and pausing when needed. In contrast, some babies fed from a bottle, particularly those younger than four months, struggle to keep up with the rapid flow of milk. If your baby seems to be gulping down the milk as fast as he can, you may think he is very hungry, but actually he may be swallowing quickly just to avoid choking. You may see signs that the baby is feeling stressed: He may tense up, and his eyes may open wide. Milk may leak from the corners of his mouth. He may try to pull away from the bottle or "shut down," pretending to fall asleep in an attempt to end the feeding. A baby who manages to chug his milk from a bottle may end up taking more than he needs.

You (or whoever is feeding the baby) can avoid this problem by making sure that the baby is comfortable, that he can pause to take a breath between swallows, and that he can end the feeding himself when he has had enough. This is known as "baby-led" or "paced" bottle-feeding. Use a slow-flow nipple, and sit the baby almost upright. Touch the bottle nipple to the baby's lips to stimulate him to open his mouth wide, as he does when he seeks out the breast. Then place the nipple in his mouth. Hold the bottle horizontally to slow the flow of milk through the nipple. There will be air in the nipple, but try not to worry about the baby swallowing it; you can burp him periodically. If he is sucking without pause but showing facial signals of stress, lower the bottle while keeping it in his mouth. This will give the baby the chance to rest and to begin sucking again when he is ready. When the baby stops sucking, do not jiggle the nipple in his mouth to get him to resume. Assume that he has had enough even if there is still milk in the bottle. You can view Jessica Barton's video on "Paced Bottle-Feeding for the Breast-Fed Baby" at www.youtube.com/watch?v=UH4T70OSzGs.

Some final words on bottle-feeding: Never prop a bottle for a young baby or allow an older baby to bottle-feed himself. A baby needs an adult in close contact not only to monitor the amount of milk taken but also to provide the pleasure of her arms and attention.

RETURNING TO WORK OR SCHOOL

Not so long ago, a new mother planning to return to work might never have considered nursing her baby or would have decided to wean near the end of her maternity leave. Today, with the growing number of working women and the increasing awareness of the many benefits breastfeeding offers, more and more mothers are choosing to nurse their babies while continuing with their careers.

Your extra efforts to continue nursing are well worth your while. The cost of formula aside, breastfed babies are generally healthier. The less your baby is sick, the less time you must spend away from work or school. Nursing also saves you time and energy, which is especially important when you are combining the responsibilities of employment and family. Perhaps most important, nursing helps you maintain the close, loving relationship you have with your baby. Many mothers who work outside the home or attend school feel that breastfeeding offers emotional compensation for the hours that must be spent apart. The security of your breast comforts the baby and helps make the time you are together special and rewarding for both of you.

Work Options

Although there may be no question in your mind that you will be returning to work or school after your baby is born, you are lucky if you have some flexibility in determining the length of your maternity leave. Your time at home after giving birth is important for both you and the baby: It is the time in which you will get to know each other and form a special bond. It will also be a time for you to rest and recover from the physical stress of the birth process. Some women need a little while, and some need a long while, before they are ready to add the demands of work or school. Breastfeeding experts have noted that mothers who stay home for 16 weeks or longer experience fewer difficulties maintaining their milk supply once back at work.

Because you cannot know just how you will feel after you deliver, explore what options may be open to you ahead of time. Depending on your financial situation and your work demands, you may be able to arrange for an extended leave, beyond the usual six to eight weeks. In 1993, the United States enacted the Family Medical Leave Act (FMLA), which requires employers with 50 or more employees to allow 12 weeks unpaid leave each year for any employee who needs to care for a dependent. Taking unpaid leave may be helpful to you, or it may not be financially feasible. You may be able instead to arrange to work at home, return to work part-time, or share your job with another person. Each of these options has worked well for many mothers. If you are a student, perhaps you can take fewer classes for a term or take some classes online.

Part-time work offers many advantages to the nursing mother. Fewer hours apart means fewer missed feedings, lower child-care costs, and generally less stress for both mother and baby.

An employer also benefits by agreeing to shorter hours. Replacing an employee is time-consuming and costly, especially if she has special skills that are an asset to the organization. Besides, many employers find part-time employees to be just as productive as those who work full-time, if not more so. Part-timers tend to stay out sick less often, and they generally waste less time when they are at work.

You might agree to come in for fewer hours each day, or have fewer full-hour days. Both arrangements have advantages and drawbacks for the nursing mother.

Still, a somewhat flexible arrangement may be possible. With a "flextime" schedule, you might work eight hours a day but remain free to start earlier or later than normal. This system could allow you to spend a leisurely morning with the baby and perhaps get a few chores done. If your partner also has a flexible schedule, you might be able to minimize the number of hours that the baby must be left with someone else.

Some mothers arrange to take their babies to work with them. Although this is not possible for most women, it can be managed in some work settings. Another option is childcare at the work site. Some employers and employees have found this to be an ideal arrangement. If you work with other parents of infants or small children, you might together explore this possibility.

Another possibility is having the baby brought to you for nursings, or going to the baby yourself during your lunch hour. Usually, the major obstacle in having the baby come to your workplace is finding someone willing and able to bring her. If instead you'll go to the baby, you will want to find childcare as close as possible to your workplace. If you have a full hour for lunch and your baby is nearby, you may have enough time to leisurely manage travel, nursing, and eating.

PLANNING YOUR RETURN TO WORK

If you will be missing one or more feedings while you are away at work or school, you should plan to express your milk. This will help prevent engorgement and, more important, maintain your milk supply. The milk you express can be used later to feed your baby while you are away. See Chapter 5 for information on

- expression methods,
- types and brands of pumps,
- other purchases you may want to consider,
- pumping at home in preparation for your return to work or school,
- expressing milk in the workplace,
- increasing your milk supply,
- storing your expressed milk, and
- feeding your milk to the baby.

Besides finding a caregiver for your baby, choosing a pump, and learning to use it, your main task in planning a return to work is to identify a place to express your milk. For some mothers, this can be difficult. Working out this problem ahead of time can help reduce the stress once you are back at work or school.

In 2010, the Affordable Care Act amended the Fair Labor Standards Act to require employers with 50 or more employees to provide a "reasonable" break time for employees who need to express breast milk for their nursing children. They are required to provide this until the baby turns one year old. Employers must also provide a place for the employee to express the milk, other than a bathroom. This area must be shielded from view and free from intrusion from co-workers and the public.

Employers are not required to pay an employee for any work time spent for expressing breast milk. However, employees who already receive compensated breaks may use that time to express milk.

State laws override this federal law if they provide greater protections to employees. For example, some states may mandate providing paid break time or providing break time beyond the baby's first birthday. As of this writing, 24 states, the District of Columbia, and Puerto Rico have additional laws regarding breastfeeding in the workplace. If you have additional questions about this law, visit www.usbreastfeeding.org.

Ideally, the place where you will pump will be quiet and private, with few distractions. Because many popular pumps operate with a battery pack, you may not need an electric outlet. A women's lounge with a comfortable chair (and preferably a sink and a refrigerator) or your own private office might be perfect. Other possibilities include a lighted storage closet, a conference room, or a borrowed office. If your workplace has a break room that both male and female employees use, you might be able to schedule your break at a time when you can have the privacy you need.

You may find that the only available place for you to express milk is a bathroom. It may be adequate as long as it is clean and has a chair, or room for one to be brought in.

If your job requires a good deal of travel, you can express milk in your car or in comfortable restrooms on your route.

If you are returning to school, you may be able to find a private place there as well. Locker rooms, empty classrooms, and health centers are all possibilities.

You may have an easier time identifying a pumping place if other mothers have worked this out before you. Otherwise, you may need to make a special trip to your workplace or school to search out a site that could work for you.

Once you're sure of your rights, discuss your need for a pumping place with your supervisor or human resources manager. Do so by letter or email if you fear your boss will be uncomfortable discussing your breasts in person or over the phone. You might consider including a letter from your doctor or your baby's doctor (you can find a letter to download and have your physician sign at www.workandpump.com/ letter.htm). You might also refer your boss to two good sources of information about why employers should support nursing mothers in the workplace. One is the United States Breastfeeding Committee website, at www.usbreastfeeding.org; the other is the Office on Women's Health website, at www.womenshealth.gov. The latter site includes an excellent printable brochure called "The Business Case for Breastfeeding." Your boss may be more supportive knowing that by facilitating breastfeeding the company will be reducing medical costs, absenteeism, and employee turnover.

Your boss may want to know whether you'll be using work time to express your milk. Your regular breaks will probably be adequate. If you need extended breaks, you can deduct the time from your total hours or make it up at the end of the day.

You will also need a cool place to store your milk. Investigate whether a refrigerator is available. Note that breast milk is not considered by the U.S. Centers for Disease Control and Prevention (CDC) or the Occupational Safety and Health Administration (OSHA) to be a "biohazardous material," which would require storage in a refrigerator where no other food is kept. If it makes you or your co-workers more comfortable, of course, you can put your milk containers in an opaque sack or lunch bag.

If no refrigerator is available, you can plan to bring a small cooler with plastic ice packs inside. Milk stays cold for several hours in a cooler, which is also handy for transporting milk home or to the caregiver's.

INSTRUCTIONS FOR THE CAREGIVER

Whether your baby goes to day care, has a nanny, or stays with a friend or family member, it is important for you to communicate exactly what you expect. Reviewing your expectations with your baby's caregiver before your return to work can help prevent misunderstandings and disappointments. There may be many other matters that you wish to discuss, but when it comes to feedings, the first and most important rule should be that your baby always be held while being fed. Your baby may be capable of holding his own bottle, but he would miss out on important human contact if he were left to feed himself.

Your baby's caregiver will also need to know how to defrost and warm breast milk. You can write these instructions out so she won't forget them. Be sure to say what to do with milk that is left in the bottle.

Give the caregiver general guidelines on how often the baby should be fed and how much he will need at each feeding. When a baby fusses, it's easiest to respond first with a bottle. Without guidelines, a caregiver may feed a baby as much milk during an eight- to ten-hour period as he would normally take over an entire day! Explain that most breastfed babies need to be fed about every two to three hours and need no more than 1½ ounces per hour. This means, for example, that a typical baby needs about 3 ounces every two hours or 4½ ounces every three hours. You might also describe to your care provider how to feed your baby using "paced" bottle-feeding (see page 157).

Underfeeding can become a problem, too. A baby who enjoys sucking on his fingers or a pacifier much of the time may not give clear feeding cues and end up not taking enough milk during the time mother and baby are apart. The general rule of 3 ounces every two to two and a half hours should prevent this.

Ask the caregiver to plan feedings so that the baby is hungry when you return for him. This generally means that the baby's last bottle-feeding of the day should be two to three hours before you are expected. If the baby seems hungry after that, the caregiver might offer a partial feeding.

When you pick up the baby at the caregiver's house, you can leave milk, labeled with the date, in her refrigerator for the next day. Fresh refrigerated milk is best for the baby, since it retains more antibodies than frozen milk. If the milk will not be used during the following three days, it should be frozen.

A few caregivers express concern about the safety of handling breast milk; they apparently fear that diseases might be transmitted through it. You can assure your caregiver that, according to the CDC and OSHA, people handling and feeding breast milk need not wear rubber gloves nor store the milk in a refrigerator where no other foods are kept.

REFRIGERATED MILK

Use refrigerated milk within 72 hours. Take the milk out of the refrigerator just before the feeding. Over 5 to 10 minutes, warm the milk to room temperature in a container of warm water. Do not warm the milk in a microwave or on the stove. If the baby doesn't take all the milk at once, you can return the leftover milk to the refrigerator and use it at the next feeding.

FROZEN MILK

Use milk within three months if it has been stored in the freezer compartment of a refrigerator. Milk stored in a deep freezer is good for six months or longer. Always use the oldest milk first. Thaw the milk either in the refrigerator, where it can remain for up to 24 hours, or in water just before feeding, gradually increasing the temperature to warm. Do not defrost the milk in a microwave or on the stove. Whatever milk the baby does not take must be discarded. Breast milk should not be refrozen.

BACK AT WORK

Once you are back at work, you will discover what routines work best for you, your baby, and your milk supply. It will help if you can nurse as much as possible when you are with the baby and express milk frequently when you are apart. Some mothers keep their milk plentiful by encouraging their babies to nurse frequently during the evening and night. You may find that bringing the baby to bed with you, if she isn't already there, and nursing an hour or so before getting up works well. Nursing twice in the morning before you leave the baby is ideal. You can nurse again just before you leave home or when you arrive at the caregiver's. While you are at work, try to express milk about as often as you would be nursing at home. Ideally, if you will be missing three feedings, you should express milk three times. Your goal should be to drain both breasts as completely as possible, by either nursing or expressing milk, at least seven times in each 24 hours.

While some mothers need to concentrate on the task at hand while they are expressing milk, others take this time to simply relax, and some mothers use the time to get work done. For mothers who use a pump, pumping both breasts at once not only increases the amount of milk collected but cuts the time of expression in half. You can probably learn how to hold both flanges to your breasts using just one arm so you can use your free hand to massage your breasts, turn pages of a book or magazine, or hold the phone to your ear. You might also try a "pumping bra," which holds both flanges in place so that a mother can express her milk and have both hands free.

Label your milk with your baby's name and the date before storing it in a refrigerator or placing it in a cooler for transport.

Some mothers leak milk while they are at work. You may need to wear thick pads in your bra; keep an extra supply of them with you. Or try silicone nursing pads, which don't absorb milk but instead apply pressure to prevent leakage. Some mothers prefer to use plastic breast shells to keep their clothes dry. Although they usually serve the purpose, these cups can also encourage further leaking. Finally, wearing printed blouses or keeping an extra jacket or sweater at work will help hide any wetness.

After work, you may want to nurse when you arrive at the caregiver's, before going home. Many mothers find this provides a welcome opportunity to relax and talk with the caregiver about the baby's day.

Some women find that they are unable to express as much milk as they would like, especially after three to four months postpartum. At this point you may notice a drop in the amount you can pump, but this doesn't necessarily mean you can't meet your baby's needs. Many women overproduce in the first few months; after about four months, milk supply is determined by demand. If you had previously been pumping excess milk, you might now find yourself producing only as much as the baby drinks while you are away. This means that your body has adjusted to the baby's needs. Normal milk production is about 1½ ounces per hour, so if three hours have passed since you last pumped, you should get 4 to 5 ounces combined when you pump both breasts.

If your milk production is good but your caregiver is running out of the milk you save, find out just how much milk your baby is taking while you're away. A baby in day care for eight hours needs no more than 12 ounces of milk during that period. If you are able to nurse when you drop your baby off, or shortly before that, and again when you pick her up, she needs only about 8 ounces while you're gone. Your baby is being overfed if she is taking much more than this. If the caregiver complains that she needs more milk to feed your baby, say that your doctor recommends that the baby have no more than 1½ ounces per hour. You might have the baby's caregiver try a slow-flow bottle nipple so the baby can suck for a longer period of time without taking more milk. Although babies do not require fluids in addition to breast milk, you might suggest a bottle of water to soothe your baby when she has been recently fed but is fussy, especially if you are expected to arrive shortly.

Your caregiver may say that your baby needs more milk because she is getting bigger. In fact, researchers report that the amount of breast milk needed over a 24-hour period by an exclusively breastfed baby changes little between the ages of one and six months. As they get older, babies utilize breast milk more efficiently.

If a baby begins taking less milk at home because of longer sleep stretches at night, however, she may want to make up for it with more milk during the day, at least until she begins eating solid foods. In this case, try to nurse more often in the evening and early morning.

If you think that your milk supply truly is too low, be sure to read "Increasing Your Milk Supply while Pumping," page 151.

If you follow all of the other recommendations here and on page 136 and still cannot express milk as often as necessary at work, you may find that the baby needs supplemental formula when you are away.

If you and your partner are both working, you may be too overwhelmed by chores to cuddle and enjoy the baby as much as you would like during your hours at home. Perhaps you can afford to pay someone to come every week or so to catch up on the housecleaning.

Combining nursing and working takes a great deal of time and energy. Aside from the responsibilities of your job, the baby, and the rest of your family, it is very important that you take time to care for yourself. Nursing mothers need to eat well. Although it may be tempting to skip breakfast or lunch, most women who do this find they have little energy to meet the many demands of the day. Get up a little earlier, if you must, to fix a nutritious breakfast. Bring snacks such as yogurt, cheese, nuts, and fruit to eat throughout the workday. Some mothers find that brewer's yeast gives them an energy boost and helps keep up the milk supply. To avoid constipation and plugged milk ducts, you will also need to drink plenty of fluids while you are at work. Finally, rest is essential. Most working and nursing mothers find that they must go to bed earlier than they once did. If you can, take an hour's nap just before dinner, and nap on your days at home with the baby.

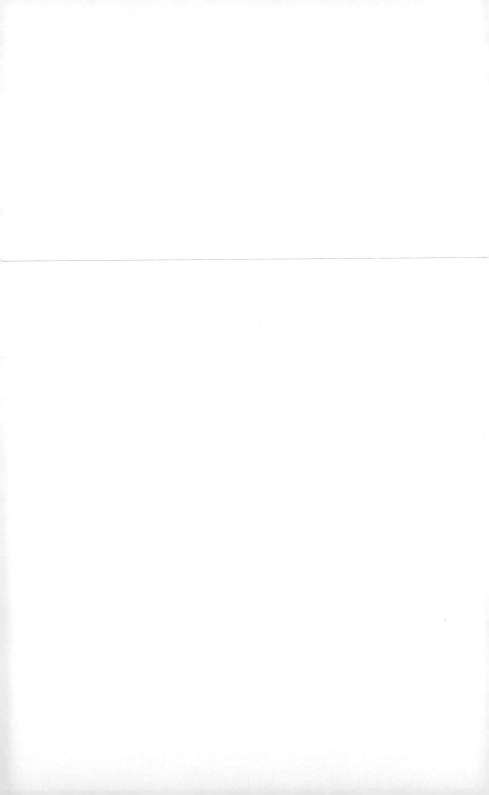

YOUR
BREASTFEEDING
DIARY

In the following pages you will find eight grids, each of which can be used as a one-day diary that helps you keep track of your baby's feedings and other important details. These diary grids are excerpted from *The Nursing Mother's Breastfeeding Diary*, © 2007, by Kathleen Huggins with Jan Ellen Brown. Because you will be nursing for more than eight days, you are encouraged to order a copy of that book, which has grids for many more days as well as inspirational quotes, space for your own journal entries, and text that suggests things to watch out for at each day. Or, if you like, you can make copies of the blank grids that follow and use those for the ninth day and all subsequent days.

Start the diary on the day your baby is born. For each day, you'll find a grid for tracking input (feedings) and output (wet and dirty diapers). The grid has space for twelve feedings per day; if you find you're nursing more frequently than this, record only the feedings that are more than just snacks.

The first column is for noting the time that the feeding started; the second is for indicating which breast you started on (L or R), so you'll know to start the following feeding on the other side. In the columns headed L and R, you can estimate the time the baby spent actively nursing—that is, sucking and swallowing—on each side (you may prefer to skip this detail). If you elect or need to express milk, record the amount you collect under "Amount Expressed." If you give the baby a full or partial feeding of formula or pumped breast milk, you can note the amount you feed in either the column headed "Breast Milk" or the one headed "Formula." Finally, in the bottom row, marked "Totals," you can total your daily amounts. This will be particularly helpful if you are pumping or feeding expressed milk or formula.

DAY AND DATE:

	TIME	START (L OR R)	MINUTES L	MINUTES R	AMOUNT EXPRESSED	SUPPLEMENT AMOUNT BREAST MILK	SUPPLEMENT AMOUNT FORMULA	OUTPUT WET	OUTPUT POOP
1									
2									
3									
4									
5									
6									
7									
8									
9									
10									
11									
12									

TOTALS:

DAY AND DATE:

| TIME | START (L OR R) | MINUTES | | AMOUNT EXPRESSED | SUPPLEMENT AMOUNT | | OUTPUT | |
		L	R		BREAST MILK	FORMULA	WET	POOP
1								
2								
3								
4								
5								
6								
7								
8								
9								
10								
11								
12								

TOTALS:

DAY AND DATE:

TIME	START (L OR R)	MINUTES		AMOUNT EXPRESSED	SUPPLEMENT AMOUNT		OUTPUT	
		L	R		BREAST MILK	FORMULA	WET	POOP
1								
2								
3								
4								
5								
6								
7								
8								
9								
10								
11								
12								

TOTALS:

DAY AND DATE:

| | TIME | START (L OR R) | MINUTES | | AMOUNT EXPRESSED | SUPPLEMENT AMOUNT | | OUTPUT | |
			L	R		BREAST MILK	FORMULA	WET	POOP
1									
2									
3									
4									
5									
6									
7									
8									
9									
10									
11									
12									

TOTALS:

DAY AND DATE: _____

| TIME | START (L OR R) | MINUTES | | AMOUNT EXPRESSED | SUPPLEMENT AMOUNT | | OUTPUT | |
		L	R		BREAST MILK	FORMULA	WET	POOP
1								
2								
3								
4								
5								
6								
7								
8								
9								
10								
11								
12								
TOTALS:								

DAY AND DATE:

| TIME | START (L OR R) | MINUTES | | AMOUNT EXPRESSED | SUPPLEMENT AMOUNT | | OUTPUT | |
		L	R		BREAST MILK	FORMULA	WET	POOP
1								
2								
3								
4								
5								
6								
7								
8								
9								
10								
11								
12								

TOTALS:

DAY AND DATE:

	TIME	START (L OR R)	MINUTES		AMOUNT EXPRESSED	SUPPLEMENT AMOUNT		OUTPUT	
			L	R		BREAST MILK	FORMULA	WET	POOP
1									
2									
3									
4									
5									
6									
7									
8									
9									
10									
11									
12									

TOTALS:

DAY AND DATE:

TIME	START (L OR R)	MINUTES		AMOUNT EXPRESSED	SUPPLEMENT AMOUNT		OUTPUT	
		L	R		BREAST MILK	FORMULA	WET	POOP
1								
2								
3								
4								
5								
6								
7								
8								
9								
10								
11								
12								

TOTALS:

APPENDIX

DETERMINING BABIES' MILK NEEDS DURING THE FIRST SIX WEEKS

Ten-Percent Weight Loss

A newborn should lose less than 10 percent of her birth weight before she begins to gain weight. Find your baby's birth weight in the left column of the table. Look at the figure across from your baby's birth weight in the right column. If your baby weighs this amount or less, you'll want to compare her milk needs (see the following sections of this appendix) with your milk production, and take steps to increase her milk intake.

BIRTH WEIGHT (IN POUNDS-OUNCES)	10% LESS	BIRTH WEIGHT (IN POUNDS-OUNCES)	10% LESS	BIRTH WEIGHT (IN POUNDS-OUNCES)	10% LESS
4-8	4-2	5-14	5-5	7-4	6-8
4-9	4-2.5	5-15	5-5.5	7-5	6-9
4-10	4-3	6-0	5-6	7-6	6-10
4-11	4-3.5	6-1	5-7	7-7	6-11
4-12	4-4	6-2	5-8	7-8	6-12
4-13	4-5	6-3	5-9	7-9	6-13
4-14	4-6	6-4	5-10	7-10	6-14
4-15	4-7	6-5	5-11	7-11	6-15
5-0	4-8	6-6	5-12	7-12	7-0
5-1	4-9	6-7	5-13	7-13	7-0.5
5-2	4-10	6-8	5-14	7-14	7-1
5-3	4-11	6-9	5-14.5	7-15	7-2
5-4	4-12	6-10	5-15	8-0	7-3
5-5	4-12.5	6-11	6-0	8-1	7-4
5-6	4-13	6-12	6-1	8-2	7-5
5-7	4-14	6-13	6-2	8-3	7-6
5-8	4-15	6-14	6-3	8-4	7-7
5-9	5-0	6-15	6-4	8-5	7-8
5-10	5-1	7-0	6-5	8-6	7-9
5-11	5-2	7-1	6-6	8-7	7-9.5
5-12	5-3	7-2	6-7	8-8	7-10
5-13	5-4	7-3	6-7.5	8-9	7-11

BIRTH WEIGHT (IN POUNDS-OUNCES)	10% LESS	BIRTH WEIGHT (IN POUNDS-OUNCES)	10% LESS	BIRTH WEIGHT (IN POUNDS-OUNCES)	10% LESS
8-10	7-12	9-12	8-12	10-14	9-13
8-11	7-13	9-13	8-13	10-15	9-13.5
8-12	7-14	9-14	8-14	11-0	9-14.5
8-13	7-15	9-15	8-15	11-1	9-15
8-14	8-0	10-0	9-0	11-2	10-0
8-15	8-1	10-1	9-1	11-3	10-1
9-0	8-2	10-2	9-2	11-4	10-2
9-1	8-2.5	10-3	9-3	11-5	10-3
9-2	8-3	10-4	9-4	11-6	10-4
9-3	8-4	10-5	9-4.5	11-7	10-5
9-4	8-5	10-6	9-5	11-8	10-5.5
9-5	8-6	10-7	9-6	11-9	10-6.5
9-6	8-7	10-8	9-7	11-10	10-7.5
9-7	8-8	10-9	9-8	11-11	10-8
9-8	8-9	10-10	9-9	11-12	10-9
9-9	8-10	10-11	9-10	11-13	10-10
9-10	8-10.5	10-12	9-11	11-14	10-11
9-11	8-11.5	10-13	9-12	11-15	10-12

BABIES' MILK NEEDS DURING THE FIRST FIVE DAYS

Find your baby's age in the left column. At right is the amount of milk he needs at each of eight daily feedings.

BABY'S AGE, IN HOURS	MILK NEEDED PER FEEDING	
	in Milliliters	in Ounces
24–48	15	1/2
48–72	20	2/3
72–96	30	1
96–120	45	1 1/2

BABIES' MILK NEEDS FROM FIVE DAYS TO SIX WEEKS OF AGE

Follow these steps to determine how much milk your baby needs.

Step 1. Weigh the baby naked, on an accurate scale, at least one hour after a feeding. Find the baby's weight in kilograms in the chart below. If the baby weighs 7 pounds, 5 ounces, for example, look down the column headed "7" and across the row headed "5." The baby's weight in kilograms is 3.317.

Ounces	\multicolumn{11}{c}{POUNDS}

Ounces	4	5	6	7	8	9	10	11	12	13	14
0	1.814	2.268	2.722	3.175	3.629	4.082	4.536	4.990	5.443	5.897	6.350
1	1.843	2.296	2.750	3.203	3.657	4.111	4.564	5.018	5.471	5.925	6.379
2	1.871	2.325	2.778	3.232	3.685	4.139	4.593	5.046	5.500	5.953	6.407
3	1.899	2.353	2.807	3.260	3.714	4.167	4.621	5.075	5.528	5.982	6.435
4	1.928	2.381	2.835	3.289	3.742	4.196	4.649	5.103	5.557	6.010	6.464
5	1.956	2.410	2.863	3.317	3.770	4.224	4.678	5.131	5.585	6.038	6.492
6	1.984	2.438	2.892	3.345	3.799	4.252	4.706	5.160	5.613	6.067	6.520
7	2.013	2.466	2.920	3.374	3.827	4.281	4.734	5.188	5.642	6.095	6.549
8	2.041	2.495	2.948	3.402	3.856	4.309	4.763	5.216	5.670	6.123	6.577
9	2.070	2.523	2.977	3.430	3.884	4.337	4.791	5.245	5.698	6.152	6.605
10	2.098	2.551	3.005	3.459	3.912	4.366	4.819	5.273	5.727	6.180	6.634
11	2.126	2.580	3.033	3.487	3.941	4.394	4.848	5.301	5.755	6.209	6.662
12	2.155	2.608	3.062	3.515	3.969	4.423	4.876	5.330	5.783	6.237	6.690
13	2.183	2.637	3.090	3.544	3.997	4.451	4.904	5.358	5.812	6.265	6.719
14	2.211	2.665	3.118	3.572	4.026	4.479	4.933	5.386	5.840	6.294	6.747
15	2.240	2.693	3.147	3.600	4.054	4.508	4.961	5.415	5.868	6.322	6.776

Step 2. To determine the approximate amount of milk a baby needs in a 24-hour period, multiply the baby's weight in kilograms by 6, and round the result to the nearest whole number.

Example: 3.317 kilograms × 6 = 19.902 ounces

If the baby weighs 3.317 kilograms, she needs approximately 20 ounces of milk per day.

Step 3. Calculate how much milk the baby needs at each feeding. Divide the amount of milk the baby needs daily by the number of times she nurses in each 24-hour period.

Example: 20 ounces ÷ 8 = 2½ ounces

If the baby needs 20 ounces of milk per day and nurses eight times per day, she needs 2½ ounces of milk at each feeding.

If the baby is taking eight feedings per day, however, you can skip step 2, and instead multiply the baby's current weight in kilograms by 22.5. The result will be the amount of milk the baby needs at each feeding in milliliters.

Example: 3.317 kilograms x 22.5 = 74.6325 milliliters

A baby weighing 3.317 kilograms needs approximately 75 milliliters of milk per feeding. To find this amount in ounces, divide by 30.

Example: 75 milliliters ÷ 30 = 2½ ounces

The baby in our example needs 2½ ounces of milk at each of eight daily feedings.

If the baby is taking nine feedings every 24 hours, you can find how much milk she needs at each feeding by multiplying her weight in kilograms by 20.

Example: 3.317 kilograms x 20 = 66.34 milliliters

The baby weighing 3.317 kilograms and nursing nine times per day needs about 66 milliliters of milk at each feeding.

Example: 66 milliliters ÷ 30 = 21/5 ounces

Since 30 milliliters equals 1 ounce, the baby needs $2^1/_5$ ounces of milk nine times per day.

SUGGESTED SUPPLMENTAL READING

Balaskas, Janet. *Active Birth: The New Approach to Giving Birth Naturally,* rev. ed. Boston: Harvard Common Press, 1992.

Bumgarner, Norma Jane. *Mothering Your Nursing Toddler.* Shaumburg, IL: La Leche League International, 2000.

Flower, Hilary. *Adventures in Tandem Nursing: Breastfeeding during Pregnancy and Beyond.* Shaumburg, IL: La Leche League International, 2003.

Fraiberg, Selma H. *The Magic Years.* New York: Charles Scribner's Sons, 1996.

Gromada, Karen Kerkhoff. *Mothering Multiples.* Shaumburg, IL: La Leche League International, 2007.

Huggins, Kathleen. *The Expectant Parents' Companion: Simplifying What to Do, Buy, or Borrow for an Easy Life with Baby.* Boston: Harvard Common Press, 2006.

Huggins, Kathleen. *The Nursing Mother's Companion,* 7th ed. Boston: Harvard Common Press, 2017.

Huggins, Kathleen, and Jan Ellen Brown. *The Nursing Mother's Companion Breastfeeding Diary.* Boston: Harvard Common Press, 2010.

Huggins, Kathleen, and Jan Ellen Brown. *25 Things Every Nursing Mother Needs to Know.* Boston: Harvard Common Press, 2009.

Huggins, Kathleen, and Linda Ziedrich. *The Nursing Mother's Guide to Weaning,* rev. ed. Boston: Harvard Common Press, 2007.

Karp, Harvey. *The Happiest Baby on the Block.* New York: Bantam Books, 2003.

Kleiman, Karen R., and Valerie D. Raskin. *This Isn't What I Expected: Overcoming Postpartum Depression.* New York: Bantam Books, 2013.

Kropp, Tori. *The Joy of Pregnancy: The Complete, Candid, and Reassuring Companion for Parents-to-Be.* Boston: Harvard Common Press, 2008.

McKenna, James. *Sleeping with Your Baby: A Parent's Guide to Cosleeping.* Washington, DC: Platypus Media, 2007.

Pantley, Elizabeth, and William Sears. *The No-Cry Sleep Solution.* New York: Contemporary Books, 2002.

Pryor, Gale, and Kathleen Huggins. *Nursing Mother, Working Mother,* rev. ed. Boston: Harvard Common Press, 2007.

Robertson, Laurel, Carol Flinders, and Brian Ruppenthal. *The New Laurel's Kitchen.* Berkeley, CA: Ten Speed Press, 1986.

Sears, William, Martha Sears, Robert Sears, and James Sears. *The Baby Book: Everything You Need to Know about Your Baby from Birth to Age Two,* rev. ed. Boston: Little, Brown, 2013.

Simkin, Penny. *The Birth Partner: A Complete Guide to Childbirth for Dads, Doulas, and All Other Labor Companions,* 3rd ed. Boston: Harvard Common Press, 2007.

Simkin, Penny, Janet Whalley, and Ann Keppler. *Pregnancy, Childbirth, and the Newborn: The Complete Guide.* Minnetonka, MN: Meadowbrook, 2001.

Vartabedian, Bryan. *Colic Solved: The Essential Guide to Infant Reflux and the Care of Your Crying, Difficult-to-Soothe Baby.* New York: Ballantine Books, 2007.

INDEX